PRAISE FOR . . .

THE NURSING MOTHER'S COMPANION

"A delightful, beautifully illustrated, and thoroughly practical book."

Sheila Kitzinger,
author of *The Complete Book of Pregnancy and Childbirth*

"A complete, practical, and easy-to-use guide which will help mothers prevent or solve the usual and not-so-usual breastfeeding problems. Huggins's expertise and warmth shine through every page."

Penny Simkin,
co-author of *Pregnancy, Childbirth, and the Newborn*

"With a unique format that is easy to follow, *The Nursing Mother's Companion* is a welcome addition to the growing wealth of information available to nursing mothers today."

Marian Tompson,
co-founder of La Leche League

"I loved *The Nursing Mother's Companion*. Helpful, complete, and readable, it's ideal for every nursing mother."

Michelle Harrison, M.D.,
author of *A Woman in Residence*

"Health care providers seeking a single book to which they can refer nursing mothers need look no further. *The Nursing Mother's Companion* will fill the bill."

Kathleen Auerbach, Ph.D.,
professional lactation consultant

THE NURSING MOTHER'S COMPANION

5th edition

Kathleen Huggins

Foreword by Ruth A. Lawrence

The Harvard Common Press

Boston, Massachusetts

The Harvard Common Press
535 Albany Street
Boston, Massachusetts 02118
www.harvardcommonpress.com

Printed in the United States of America

Library of Congress Cataloging-in-Publication Data

Huggins, Kathleen.
    The nursing mother's companion / Kathleen Huggins ;
foreword by Ruth A. Lawrence. -- 5th ed.
        p.   cm.
    Includes bibliographical references and index.
    ISBN 1-55832-303-1 (hc : alk. paper) --
    ISBN 1-55832-304-X (pb : alk paper)
    1. Breast feeding--Popular works.   I. Title.
RJ216.H845   2005
649'.33--dc22   2004021182

ISBN-13: 978-1-55832-304-9
ISBN-10: 1-55832-304-X

Special bulk-order discounts are available on this and other
Harvard Common Press books. Companies, organizations,
and health care providers may purchase books for premiums
or for resale, or may arrange a custom edition, by contacting
the Marketing Director at the address above.

Interior design by Cia Boynton
Cover design by Jackie Schuman
Illustrations by Susan Aldridge
Author photograph by McClain Photography
Photographs © Getty Images, except for page 231,
by Patricia Jalbert-Levine

10   9

To the nursing mothers of San Luis Obispo,
who have been my teachers

CONTENTS

FOREWORD

Centuries ago few women faced decisions about how to feed their babies: the newborn's only means of survival was mother's milk. Today, however, there are safe alternatives to nursing, and so a woman needs to think about how she wishes to feed her baby and what method is really best for them both. If she decides to nurse her baby as her ancestors did theirs, she must make an effort to learn how. Breastfeeding is the physiologic continuation of the normal reproductive cycle, and babies are born knowing how to find the nipple and to suck; their mothers, however, do not instinctively know how to nurse. Many women today have never seen a baby breastfed and have little access to experienced nursing mothers. Today's mothers have to learn what to do.

An expectant mother must first learn about alternative feeding methods so she can make an informed choice. With this book, Kathleen Huggins helps the mother through the decision-making process by providing sound information about the practical advantages of breastfeeding, its importance to a baby's health, and the very special emotional rewards it offers both mother and baby.

As a woman progresses through her pregnancy and makes preparations for her baby, she may wonder how she should also prepare for breastfeeding. Inexperienced though well-meaning friends may offer abundant but conflicting advice. This book, on the contrary, provides sensible guidelines for preparing to breastfeed, as well as an explanation of the process by which nature prepares the breast for nursing. Understanding how the breast functions prepares a woman for the physiologic changes that occur as the baby is born, the placenta is delivered, and lactation begins. It is also important that the expectant mother discuss her plans to breastfeed with her physician or midwife. The health-care provider can work together with the mother to plan the details of delivery and postpartum care to facilitate lactation.

Having made the decision to breastfeed and having prepared herself for it, a woman must learn *how* to nurse her new baby. Included here are chapters that cover methods of increasing milk production and release, or let-down, and what to do when small problems arise. The author also describes more complicated problems, though these are rare, and explains the course of treatment a doctor or midwife is likely to recommend. It is important to recognize when a situation warrants medical attention, since early appropriate management can usually minimize a problem and facilitate its resolution.

The author, who has breastfed her own children, is also a perinatal nurse who has counseled thousands of new mothers through a breastfeeding clinic and telephone hot line. With her practical experience, enhanced by her formal study of lactation, she is especially qualified to prepare this manual for mothers.

A new mother needs to be confident that she is doing the best for her baby. This book will give her the knowledge that is vital to developing that confidence. With the rich store of information herein, every mother should be able to experience the joy of breastfeeding.

Ruth A. Lawrence, M.D.
University of Rochester

PREFACE

Not long ago, a first-time nursing mother came to me about a difficulty she was having breastfeeding her baby. After we successfully resolved it, she suggested I write a book on breastfeeding that included problem-solving techniques. Although I was flattered, such a project seemed monumental. But later, as I recalled her enthusiasm, I began to consider the insights I had gained over years of assisting so many mothers, first as a maternity and newborn nurse and later after founding a breastfeeding clinic and telephone counseling service. Certainly, I was more than familiar with the common concerns of mothers who are learning to breastfeed, as well as with the occasional problems that can interfere with the development of a successful nursing relationship. The next day I wrote my rough outline.

Many excellent books had already been written on the benefits of nursing over artificial feeding methods. I set out, however, to provide mothers with a practical guide for easy reference throughout the nursing period. The first part of the book provides basic information about the breast, preparation for nursing, and nursing during the first week; the remainder of the book is intended for reading as the baby and the nursing relationship grow and develop. There are chapters on each of the three later phases of nursing—from the first week through the second month, from the second month through the sixth, and after the sixth month. Following each of these chapters is a Survival Guide—a quick yet thorough reference for almost any problem you or your baby may encounter during the phase covered. Although you may rarely need to consult the Survival Guides, I have included them to ensure that, when you do, you will be able to identify and resolve your problem as quickly as possible. Because many nursing women occasionally find themselves in need of medication, Dr. Philip Anderson has provided an appendix on drugs and their safety for the breastfed baby.

During the year I spent writing this book, I received a great deal of encouragement and guidance. I am tremendously indebted to Lynn Moen for her support along the way. I also wish to thank Penny Simkin, R.P.T., and my editor, Linda Ziedrich, for their many efforts on my behalf.

For their thoughtful review of the text I thank Marian Tompson; Andrea Herron, R.N., M.S., C.L.C.; Kathleen Rodriquez Michaelson, B.A., C.L.C.; Vicki McDonald, R.D.; Judith La Vigna; Julie Merrill, R.N.; Tom Robinson; and Kathleen Auerbach, Ph.D.

Jim Litzenburger; Vicki Gadberry, R.N., C.N.M.; Marilynn Schuster, R.N.; Kathleen Long, M.D.; and Dawn Edwards, R.N.C., are most appreciated for their encouragement as well as their friendship.

I am grateful to Donna Janetski for her commitment to this project in preparing the manuscript. My thanks also to Mike Sims for his generosity, and to Susan and Kirk Graves for their efforts.

This book would never have been possible without my husband, Brad, whose love, patience, and faith sustained me. Kate, my beautiful daughter and former nursing companion, was my inspiration throughout.

NOTE TO THE SECOND EDITION: For help in preparing this edition I would like to thank Trina Vosti, I.B.C.L.C., and Andrea VanOutryve, I.B.C.L.C. And thanks to John, my current nursing companion.

NOTE TO THE THIRD EDITION: For their extensive review of the text I wish to thank Olga Mireles, R.N., C.L.C., and Ellen ("Binky") Petok, I.B.C.L.C.

NOTE TO THE FOURTH EDITION: For their generous assistance with revisions, I thank the following women: Dayna Ravalin, R.D.; Sue Petracek, B.S. Ed.; Paula Meier D.N.Sc., R.N., F.A.A.N.; Lois D. W. Arnold, M.P.H., I.B.C.L.C.; Jan Barger, R.N., I.B.C.L.C.; Darillyn Starr; and Rachel Vireday.

NOTE TO THE FIFTH EDITION: Several years ago, on an Internet parenting site, I was lucky enough to meet "Honeysucklemama," who was nursing her first child. Rarely have I encountered such a thoughtful and supportive counselor assisting other mothers with her insightful writing. Thank you, Tricia Bulger Zack, for your fresh look at this book, as well as your support during my year of recovery from breast cancer.

I would also like to thank Patricia Donohue-Carey, L.C.C.E., C.L.E., perinatal health educator; Nancy Wight, M.D.; Jack Newman, M.D.; Lenore Goldfarb, I.B.C.L.C.; Thomas Hale, Ph.D.; James McKenna, Ph.D.; Cynthia Good Mojab, M.S., I.B.C.L.C., R.L.C.; and Darillyn Starr for reviewing portions of this new edition. My friends Binky Petok, I.B.C.L.C.; Gretta Blythe, R.N., I.B.C.L.C.; and Jan Ellen Brown, I.B.C.L.C., I thank you for your love and support.

INTRODUCTION

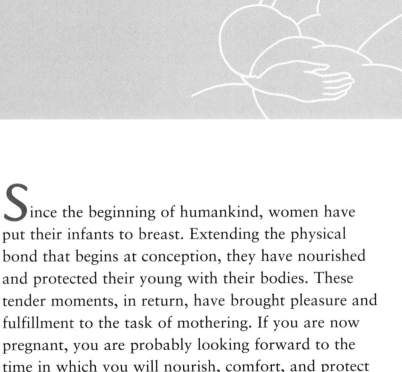

**Is Breastfeeding Really Better?
What's In It for Mom?**

Since the beginning of humankind, women have
put their infants to breast. Extending the physical
bond that begins at conception, they have nourished
and protected their young with their bodies. These
tender moments, in return, have brought pleasure and
fulfillment to the task of mothering. If you are now
pregnant, you are probably looking forward to the
time in which you will nourish, comfort, and protect
your child in the same way as others before you—at
the breast.

Perhaps you already feel committed to the idea
of nursing. For you, there is no question that you'll

breastfeed your baby. Or perhaps, like many women, you have some uncertainties, but still feel it's worth a try. Your outlook depends on many things—the value you place on breastfeeding, how your partner feels about it, how your friends have fed their babies, your lifestyle, and your feelings about yourself and your body.

You probably also have some notions about what nursing will be like. Perhaps you think it will be easy and convenient. Maybe you worry that it might not fit in with your activities and plans. You may have concerns about your ability to nurse. Probably you know of other women who tried to nurse but soon gave up. Whatever your attitudes, expectations, and concerns about breastfeeding, these may become powerful determinants in your ultimate success or failure to nurse your baby happily.

Is Breastfeeding Really Better?

You may be under the impression that the decision to breastfeed or bottle-feed is simply a matter of personal preference. Don't let anyone fool you into believing that breast milk and formula are equally good—they are not. Without a doubt, mother's milk alone promotes optimum health and development for babies. It is uniquely designed to meet the complete nutritional needs of the growing human infant. It also protects the infant against illness throughout the entire first year and beyond, as long as nursing continues.

Although babies do grow on processed infant formulas, formula manufacturers are continually challenged to include all of the nutrients in breast milk that scientists are gradually identifying as important to infant growth and development. But artificial infant milks, whether based on cow's milk or soybeans, will never be able to duplicate nature's formula. Human milk contains proteins that promote brain development and specific immunities against human illness. In contrast, cow's milk contains proteins that favor muscular growth and specific immunities to bovine disease. Babies, like all young mammals, do best with milk from their own species. Babies on a formula diet are at greater risk for illness and hospitalization. Diarrheal infections and respiratory illnesses are more frequent and serious among these babies. Formula-fed babies develop many more ear infections, which may lead to later speech and reading problems. Urinary tract infections and bacterial meningitis are more common among artificially fed infants. Formula feeding appears to be one of several factors implicated in Sudden Infant Death Syndrome (SIDS).

Formula-fed infants also have higher incidences of colic, constipation, and allergic disorders. In fact, a significant number of babies are allergic to formulas, both those based on cow's milk and those based on soy. There is also mounting evidence that artificially fed infants more often experience learning disorders and lower levels of intellectual functioning.

Bottle feeding with formula more commonly leads to overfeeding and obesity, which may well persist into childhood, adolescence, and adulthood. Tooth decay, malocclusion (improper meeting of the upper and lower teeth), and distortion of the facial muscles may also directly result from sucking on bottles.

Formula feeding may also expose a baby to toxic metals, harmful bacteria, and other environmental toxins. High levels of aluminum have been identified in most formulas. From time to time, manufacturing errors in the production of infant formulas have had serious consequences. Frequently, contamination occurs because the person preparing the baby's bottle takes too little care in handling and storing the formula and feeding equipment, or in mixing the formula with water. Babies have suffered lead poisoning when their formulas have been mixed with tap water high in lead content. Water pollution is a potential problem even if the water is purchased in a sealed bottle.

Some studies suggest that the benefits of breastfeeding over bottle feeding extend into adulthood. Breastfed babies have lower cholesterol levels and less coronary artery disease, on average, when they become adults. Breastfeeding is also protective against chronic digestive disorders, such as Crohn's Disease and ulcerative colitis. Although asthma rates are not significantly different between breastfed and non-breastfed babies, there is a lower rate of asthma in adults who were breastfed. Breastfed babies also have a smaller chance of developing Type 1 (juvenile-onset) diabetes and cancer of the lymph glands. For all of these reasons, the American Academy of Pediatrics recommends that infants be offered only breast milk for the first six months after birth, and that breastfeeding continue throughout the first year and then as long as mutually desired.

Establishing a close bond and meeting the emotional needs of a child are certainly an essential part of mothering. The nursing woman is thought to produce hormones that promote a physiologic bonding between mother and child. And in what better way can a baby be nurtured, comforted, and made to feel secure than snuggled within his mother's loving arms, against the warmth of her breast? Although some rationalize that bottle-feeding mothers can capture a similar warm feeding relationship, in reality they do not. This is partly because bottle feeding doesn't require much human contact. The bottle-fed baby generally receives less stroking, caressing, and rocking than the breastfed baby. He is talked to less often and he spends more time in his crib away from his parents. Although it is unknown how prevalent the practice of propping bottles for the young infant is, probably the overwhelming majority of babies who are able to hold their own bottles become almost entirely responsible for feeding themselves.

WHAT'S IN IT FOR MOM?

Although you may already be convinced nursing is best for your baby, you may have heard it will be a bother for you. Or you may have tried nursing a baby and given up because of difficulties. Either way, you may worry that breastfeeding will be hard, inconvenient, embarrassing, or even disgusting. This book will put those fears to rest.

Expectant mothers often hear stories about women who tried to nurse their babies but failed. Perhaps you know women who claim that they didn't produce enough milk, that it wasn't rich enough, that their milk supply dried up one day, that their milk didn't agree with their baby, or that the baby suddenly decided he wanted a bottle instead. You may even have heard that women with small breasts or those who are "nervous types" aren't able to nurse. Maybe you put no stock in these common stories, and believe instead that because nursing a baby is natural it must be easy. Sometimes it isn't. Today close to half of all mothers who start out nursing their babies give it up within the first six weeks. The reason for this failure is rarely that the mother is unable to produce enough milk. Typically it is because she is alone in her efforts to nurse. All too many new mothers know little about the nursing process and the breastfed infant, have little or no guidance, and lack support while they are learning. Although breastfeeding is natural, it is not instinctive—it must be learned.

The Nursing Mother's Companion will tell you what you need to know to breastfeed your baby. This doesn't mean that you must sit down and read this entire book before you can begin nursing. The chapters are organized chronologically, so you can read one at a time as your baby grows. If you encounter a problem along the way, use the Survival Guides for reference.

Mothers who plan to return to work often worry whether they will be able to continue nursing. Today, a growing number of women are combining motherhood, nursing, and working, and doing it quite successfully, thanks to recent advances in milk collection and storage equipment. Having a healthy baby is especially important to a working mother, and breastfed babies are sick less often. And after several hours spent apart, moreover, nursing becomes a loving reunion between a working mother and her child (see Chapter 5).

You may have heard that nursing can be painful. Normally, women find it comfortable and pleasurable. Some women worry about developing sore nipples during the early days of nursing, but most soreness can be avoided by correctly positioning the baby at the breast (see "Positioning at the Breast," page 30). You may have also heard that babies sometimes bite their mothers while nursing. When a baby is sucking, his tongue covers his lower gums and teeth so he cannot bite. Still, some babies do occasionally bite at the end of feeding, usually during a period of teething. Most babies learn very quickly not to do this.

Although the health of an infant and the emotional benefits of breastfeeding are certainly reason enough to nurse, mothers frequently have other motives.

Maybe you think that breastfeeding mothers are too "tied down." In fact, experienced nursing mothers boast about the ease and convenience of breastfeeding. They are often quick to add that information, guidance, support, and reassurance were essential at the start. After the first few weeks, however, nursing a baby simplifies life considerably.

Most experienced nursing mothers are grateful they don't have to shop for formula and prepare bottles. It's difficult to believe that getting up at night to fix a bottle is more convenient than pulling the baby to the breast and dozing off again. Outings with a nursing baby mean not having to cart around formula, bottles, and nipples wherever you go. Just because the breastfed baby is easy to take along doesn't mean she can't be left behind; you can leave milk for your infant at times the two of you must be apart.

When anticipating nursing, some women worry about modesty. Although we all know making milk is the natural function of our breasts, most of us feel embarrassed about exposing them. At first you may be more comfortable nursing in private, but most women find that, with a little time and experience, nursing in the presence of others can be discreet and comfortable. Techniques for discreet nursing are discussed in "Taking the Baby Along," page 169.

Many women worry about how they will look after they have had a baby. The fat you accumulate during pregnancy is intended for caloric reserves while nursing. Although vigorous dieting is not a

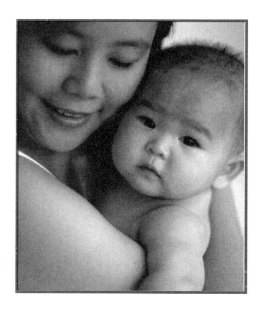

There's no pleasure to equal watching your baby grow from the nourishment of your own body.

good idea during the nursing period, most mothers find that they gradually lose weight while they are breastfeeding, so long as they are not overeating. Women who formula-feed their babies may have a much harder time losing the fat they gained during pregnancy.

Some women fear that breastfeeding will ruin the appearance of their breasts. Pregnancy typically causes the breasts to enlarge, and sometimes to develop stretch marks. During the first few months of nursing, women whose breasts are normally small or medium-sized generally find them to be bigger. Women whose breasts are normally large can usually expect them to stay about the same size as they were late in pregnancy. As the baby gets older and begins nursing less often, most women notice their breasts reduce in size. At weaning, the breasts typically appear smaller still and somewhat droopy, but within six months they generally resume their usual size and shape. Whether you nurse or not, however, you may notice a change in the firmness of your breasts after you have a baby. Childbearing, not nursing, along with age and heredity are the major determinants of the breasts' ultimate appearance.

Breastfeeding actually has beneficial effects on a woman's body. Many studies report lower rates of ovarian cancer and premenopausal breast cancer among women who have breastfed, and it appears that the risk of cancer decreases the longer a woman nurses. There is some evidence, too, that nursing offers protection against osteoporosis (brittle bones), which can occur later in life. And breastfeeding generally lengthens the time before menstrual periods resume. Most nursing women find they don't have a menstrual cycle for several months to two years after delivery, so long as they are nursing frequently.

All nursing mothers appreciate the money they save by not buying formula. Mothers committed to providing their children with wholesome, natural foods see breast milk as a sound beginning. Some mothers are repelled by the smell and taste of many formula preparations, not to mention the unpleasant odor of the bowel movements and spit-up milk of the formula-fed baby, and the stains formula may leave on clothing.

Mothers who nurse do so not only because they want the very best nourishment and protection for their babies and because they personally derive many practical benefits from breastfeeding, but simply because they enjoy the experience. The loving relationship established between mother and infant at the breast is emotionally fulfilling and pleasurable. You'll know no greater reward as a mother than witnessing your child grow from your body—first in the womb, and then at the breast.

1 Looking Forward: Preparations during Pregnancy

Learning about Breastfeeding
Ensuring the Purest Milk
Your Breasts
Planning for the First Days
Planning for the First Weeks

You may have decided to nurse your baby long before you became pregnant. Or perhaps you have just begun to consider breastfeeding. Although nourishing a baby at the breast is natural, many new mothers are surprised to find it is a learned skill—one that usually takes several weeks to master.

Success at nursing often depends upon a woman's confidence and commitment. You can develop your confidence by learning as much as possible about breastfeeding ahead of time. You can strengthen your commitment to nurse by developing a strong support system for yourself.

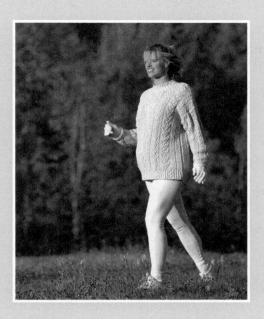

LEARNING ABOUT BREASTFEEDING

Generations ago, most new mothers turned to their own mothers for support and guidance on breastfeeding. Unfortunately, few women today can do this. For many, the art of breastfeeding is learned alone—by trial and error. All too often this leads to frustration and discouragement.

There are several ways you can learn about nursing ahead of time. Reading about it is certainly beneficial. In some communities, breastfeeding classes are offered. Expectant mothers are also most welcome to attend La Leche League meetings, which are held monthly in most areas. La Leche League is the organization of nursing mothers whose purpose is to support breastfeeding worldwide. In some areas, other groups, such as the Nursing Mothers Counsel, provide classes and telephone counseling for pregnant and nursing women. These groups are listed in Appendix A. In addition, hospitals, county health departments, and WIC (Women, Infants, and Children Supplemental Nutrition) programs may sponsor prenatal breastfeeding classes. See Appendix A, page 241, for more information about WIC.

Another excellent way to learn about breastfeeding is to spend time with women who are nursing their babies. It may be that you have never seen, close up, a mother and baby breastfeeding. Most nursing mothers will delight in your interest, and one or two may become good sources of information and support for you in the days to come. Be sure to ask them about their first weeks of nursing. Most likely you will hear of a variety of experiences, and perhaps you will develop a sense of what the early period of breastfeeding can be like.

ENSURING THE PUREST MILK

A mother may occasionally wonder if her milk is entirely safe for her child. Most frequently, this concern arises because she needs to take medication. Although most medications pass into the breast milk, the vast majority pass in only small amounts and are considered safe for the nursing infant. A comprehensive guide to drugs in breast milk can be found in Appendix C. If you can't find the information you're looking for there, call the University of California, San Diego, Drug Information Service at 900-226-7536 (consultation costs $4.00 for the first minute and $2.50 for each additional minute; calls average one to three minutes each).

More and more questions have arisen about the environmental pollutants we are exposed to, such as insecticides and other toxic chemicals. Many of these substances are stored in fatty tissues of the body, and, as a result, small amounts may be detected in breast milk. Experts on the subject, however, have been unable to identify any risks to the baby from such amounts, and most believe that the nutritional and immunological benefits of breast milk far outweigh the possible risks of environmental pollutants. Sadly, our children receive even greater exposure to some of these chemicals in the womb than they do at the breast.

If you want to minimize your baby's exposure to toxic chemicals, follow these guidelines during pregnancy and as long as you are breastfeeding:

- Stop using pesticides in the home, in the garden, and on pets.
- Avoid exposure to organic solvents, which are in paints, furniture strippers, gasoline fumes, non-water-based glues, nail polish, and

dry-cleaning fumes. Air dry-cleaned clothes outdoors before wearing them, and avoid permanently moth-proofed garments.

- Adopt a diet low in animal fat, including butterfat.

- Avoid eating fish species that have been found to have high levels of mercury and PCB, including shark, swordfish, and king mackerel, and fish caught in contaminated waters, especially the Great Lakes. The U.S. Food and Drug Administration says that pregnant women can safely eat 12 ounces per week of all other types of cooked fish, but recommends limiting consumption of grouper, martin, and orange roughy. The Environmental Working Group is even more conservative; this nonprofit organization suggests also completely avoiding fresh tuna, sea bass, Gulf Coast oysters, marlin, halibut, pike, walleye, white croaker, and largemouth bass, and eating no more than one serving a month of canned tuna, mahi mahi, blue mussels, Eastern oysters, cod, pollock, Great Lakes salmon, Gulf Coast blue crab, wild channel catfish, and lake whitefish. Safe fish and shellfish, with mercury levels lower than .2 parts per million, include farmed trout, farmed catfish, fish sticks, shrimp, pollock, wild Pacific salmon, haddock, summer-caught flounder, croaker, clams, flatfish, mid-Atlantic blue crab, freshwater sport fish, and scallops. Check with your state or local health department about the safety of local species.

- Carefully wash or peel fresh fruit and vegetables.

- Avoid crash diets, which can increase the excretion of toxic substances into breast milk.

- If you work with chemicals, ask your doctor to refer you to specialist who can advise you about their safety.

YOUR BREASTS

During pregnancy many changes occur in your breasts in preparation for nourishing your baby. Initially, you probably noticed they were more full and tender than usual. Their increasing size during the first few months of pregnancy is caused by the development of the milk-making structures within them. With this growth the blood flow to the breasts increases, and veins in the breasts may become clearly visible. Some women develop stretch marks on their breasts like the ones that can occur on the abdomen during pregnancy.

The nipple and the area around the nipple, the areola, may double in size and deepen in color; this darkening may serve as a visual cue to the newborn. Also during this time, small glands located in the areola, known as Montgomery's tubercles, become pronounced. Their function is to secrete an antibacterial lubricant that keeps the nipple moist and protected during pregnancy and breast-feeding. This is why soaps and special creams are unnecessary in caring for your breasts, and may even be harmful: soaps remove the breast's natural lubricant, and creams may interfere with its antibacterial action.

The nipples often become more sensitive during pregnancy in preparation for nursing. Some women find that their nipples are overly sensitive and even hurt when touched. This sensitivity diminishes as pregnancy advances; it should not make breastfeeding uncomfortable. Other women enjoy the sensitivity and feel great pleasure when their breasts are fondled during lovemaking.

By the fifth or sixth month of pregnancy, the breasts are fully capable of producing milk. Some women begin to notice drops of fluid on the nipple at this time. This fluid, known as colostrum, comes from the many tiny openings in the nipple and is the food your baby will receive during the first few days after birth. Some women do not leak colostrum, but it is there in the breasts just the same.

As women, we all receive messages about our bodies and what they "ought" to look like. These messages affect our self-image, including our feelings about our breasts and how they look. You can probably remember how you felt about your breasts as they developed in early adolescence. You may have felt proud as they grew larger and you began wearing a bra. Perhaps you were embarrassed

▶ *In pregnancy the breasts become enlarged, and veins and stretch marks may become visible.*

if they developed earlier or grew larger than the other girls'. You may have felt anxious if they took a long time to grow, or self-conscious if they were small.

Even now you may wish that your breasts were smaller or larger, fuller or less droopy. You may not resemble the women with "perfect" breasts portrayed in photographs of nursing mothers. Women with large breasts, especially, often feel insecure about nursing, fearing that their breasts will grow much larger still or leak milk excessively. Actually, large breasts seldom grow bigger after delivery, and they tend to leak less than small breasts.

Each woman's breasts are very different from all others, but the breast, regardless of size, is perfectly designed for its ultimate purpose—to nourish and nurture our children. The breasts not only provide an infant with superb nutrients for growth and development, but offer the warmth, the comfort, and the security that every growing baby needs. In this respect, they are most beautiful.

Caring for your breasts

During the last months of pregnancy, just rinse your breasts during your bath or shower. Avoid soaping them, since soaps tend to dry the nipples and the areola. If your breasts are dry or itchy, a mild cream or lotion may feel soothing, but avoid getting it on the nipple or areola.

Many women prefer to wear a supportive bra during pregnancy, although some are just as comfortable without one.

▲ *Breasts come in all sizes and shapes.*

The making and giving of milk

After the birth of your baby, colostrum is readily available for her first nursings. Colostrum is the ideal food for her first days; it is both perfect nutritionally and important for protection against infection. Milk generally appears by the second or third day, but occasionally not until the fourth or fifth.

Your body is signaled to initiate milk production with the delivery of the placenta. This causes the hormone prolactin to activate the milk-producing cells of the breast. The initial manufacture of milk occurs whether the baby nurses or not. Continued milk production is another matter. This depends on frequent and regular stimulation of the breast and the drainage of milk. The baby's sucking stimulates the nerve endings in the breast, which in turn trigger the release of the two hormones essential to milk production and release—prolactin and oxytocin.

Prolactin, as mentioned previously, activates the milk-producing cells in the breast to manufacture milk. Oxytocin is responsible for the release of the milk from the tiny sacs where the milk is made. This release is referred to as the ejection or let-down reflex. As the baby

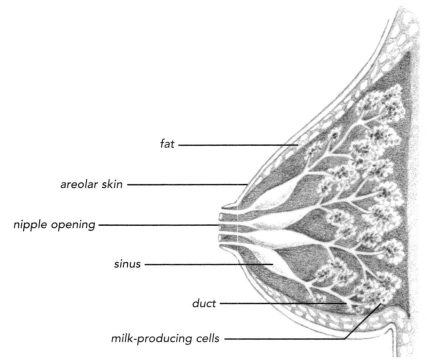

fat

areolar skin

nipple opening

sinus

duct

milk-producing cells

Cross-section of a lactating breast. ▲

nurses, the milk is propelled forward to the sinuses beneath the areola. It is the baby's job to get the milk out of the sinuses by compressing the areola with her tongue and gums as she nurses.

During the early months of her life, your baby will receive plenty of milk as long as she nurses frequently, at least eight times in 24 hours, is latched on and sucking properly, and is allowed a sufficient amount of time to complete each feeding. This is because breastfeeding works by supply and demand. The more your breasts are stimulated and emptied by the baby's sucking, the more milk you will produce.

PLANNING FOR THE FIRST DAYS

| Nipple preparation |

Often mothers who plan to breastfeed are advised to prepare their nipples during pregnancy. In fact, studies have shown that nipple "toughening" maneuvers, such as brisk rubbing or twisting, do little to prevent soreness during early breastfeeding. Whether or not they have especially sensitive skin, blondes and redheads do not generally experience any more nipple soreness than other women. Sore nipples are usually prevented by correct attachment of the baby at the breast during nursing (see "Positioning at the Breast," page 30).

If you have had one or both nipples pierced, remove the jewelry before giving birth and leave it out as long as your baby is nursing. You'll probably be able to nurse without complication, but you may find that you leak milk from the site of the piercing.

One preparation is very important during pregnancy: you should make sure your nipples can extend outward. Your baby may have difficulty grasping the breast if the nipples do not protrude enough on their own or cannot be made to protrude. Do not assume because your nipples appear to extend outward that all is well. Even if you had a breast exam earlier in your pregnancy, your nipples may not have been fully checked. Take the time to perform your own assessment.

First, look at both your nipples. They may protrude, or one or both may be flat, dimpled, folded in the center, or inverted. Next, do the "pinch test": gently squeeze just behind the nipple with your thumb and forefinger. This imitates the motion your baby will make while nursing. See how both nipples respond. If your nipples are flat, pull them outward to determine if they can lift away from the inner mass of the breast. The following chart will help you determine whether you need to take further steps to minimize initial nursing difficulties.

Usual nipple appearance	Appearance when pinched	
	Satisfactory	*Needs correction*
Protruding	Nipple stays protruded	———
Flat	Nipple can be pinched outward	Nipple moves inward or cannot be pinched outward
Dimpled or folded	Entire nipple extends outward	Nipple moves inward or flattens
Inverted	Entire nipple extends outward	Nipple extends out only slightly, remains inverted, or inverts further

When nipples need correction. The flat nipple that cannot be pinched outward, or the nipple that moves inward or flattens when compressed, is said to be "tied" to the inner breast tissue by tiny adhesions. The physical changes of pregnancy help the nipples to stand out, but one or both may still need correction. In this case, special plastic breast shells may solve the problem before breastfeeding begins.

Worn inside the bra, breast shells exert a steady but gentle pressure on the areola and cause the nipple to extend outward through the opening in the shell. This helps to loosen the adhesions beneath the nipple. Breast shells should be worn as soon as you have determined that improvement is needed, ideally from about mid-pregnancy on. They can be purchased in most maternity shops (see Appendix A for information on ordering them). Gradually work up to wearing the shells most of the day, letting comfort be your guide.

▲ *Breast shells can improve nipple shape.*

The postpartum setting

Too few mothers realize ahead of time the tremendous effect the immediate postpartum experience—in a hospital, in a birth center, or at home—can have on their breastfeeding success. It is most worthwhile to evaluate the situation you will be in after delivery to make any necessary arrangements for early nursing.

Some women have the opportunity to select among several hospitals or birth centers for their delivery. If you are making such a choice, be sure to get a recommendation from your childbirth educator or a breastfeeding counselor. She will probably know which places are most supportive of nursing mothers and infants. Even if only one hospital is available to you—and many birth attendants practice at only one—it is well worth your time to ask about the policies of the maternity unit. This will help assure that your nursing gets off to the best possible start.

Take advantage of the maternity tours, teas, and classes that most hospitals and birth centers offer, or call the postpartum unit (make sure the nurse has time to talk) to learn about policies and routines. Be sure to inquire:

- How soon after delivery will I be able to nurse? What if I have a cesarean birth?

- How often is nursing encouraged during the day and at night?

- Can the baby stay in the room with me? If not, how often and for how long will we be together?
- What assistance with breastfeeding is offered by the nursing staff?
- Does the staff avoid supplemental bottle feeding?
- Is there a lactation professional on staff?

In 1990, the United Nations Children's Fund and the World Health Organization created an award of recognition for those hospitals worldwide that have enacted ten policies to support breastfeeding mothers and babies. Hospitals that have implemented the "Ten Steps" are awarded the designation "Baby Friendly." At this writing, thirty-eight hospitals in the United States have earned baby-friendly status. When inquiring about a hospital's breastfeeding policies, ask if it has applied for the Baby-Friendly certificate. If it has, you can be assured that the nurses are committed to your breastfeeding success. If it hasn't, perhaps your inquiry will inspire the hospital to enact baby-friendly policies.

If the nurse is friendly and receptive to your questions, you might also ask which pediatricians she feels are particularly knowledgeable about breastfeeding and supportive of it.

Ideally, the maternity unit's policies encourage mothers and babies to remain together for the first few hours after birth, or at least assure that nursing takes place within the first two hours, when the baby is likely to be alert and eager to suck. Breastfeeding goes best when nursing is frequent, every one to three hours, during both day and night. "Rooming in" with the baby, at least during the day and evening, is conducive to frequent nursing and allows the mother and baby to become better acquainted before going home. Preferably, the nursing staff does not routinely give the babies water or formula supplements, as this lessens their interest in nursing and sometimes interferes with their ability to breastfeed. It can be an added bonus if the nurses enjoy assisting breastfeeding mothers or if one nurse is specifically responsible for breastfeeding counseling.

If you are planning an early discharge from a hospital or birth center, or will be delivering at home, you may also want to inquire about home visits by a nurse, lactation professional, or midwife during the first few days.

The baby's doctor

Your breastfeeding experience can be greatly influenced by your choice of physician for your child. You may want a pediatrician for your baby, or you may prefer to use a family practitioner (you may certainly choose to continue with a family practitioner who attended your baby's birth). In selecting a doctor, start by getting the names of those who are known to have a positive attitude about breastfeeding. Ask your obstetrician, midwife, childbirth educator, or a lactation professional for recommendations. You might also inquire about physicians in your area who work with nurse practitioners. These nurses have advanced education and training in well-baby care, and they usually provide mothers with extra attention and counseling on a variety of parental concerns, including breastfeeding.

Most doctors and nurse practitioners will set aside time for a preliminary visit with expectant parents. Usually this is free of charge; they realize you are "looking and choosing." Be sure to visit at least two before making a final decision, even if the first one seems nice. By all means meet the office nurse. She will often be the one who will answer your questions or concerns when you call during office hours. She can be a good resource for you, especially if she has breastfed successfully herself or has a special interest in nursing.

Let the doctor or nurse practitioner know that you are going to nurse your baby. To gauge his or her overall support of nursing mothers, ask what the recommendations would be should you experience difficulty in breastfeeding. The best pediatric practitioners offer practical assistance with breastfeeding or referrals to lactation professionals. Other practitioners provide reassuring words about feeding infant formula. Take time to discuss your preferences for feeding the baby in the hospital. If the maternity unit's policies are not ideal, ask about written orders to allow early nursing and rooming-in, and to prevent the feeding of supplements to your baby.

There may be other questions you will want to ask about the hospital or birth center, or about well-baby care. Bring a list with you so you don't forget any of them. Be sure to inquire about any necessary procedures for notifying the doctor or nurse practitioner when the baby is born. It is often said that the pediatrician takes care of the parents perhaps even more than the child. Trust your intuition when making your final choice about which pediatrician, family doctor, or nurse practitioner is right for you.

Nursing bras and pads

During the early weeks of breastfeeding, the average breast weighs three to four times as much as it did before pregnancy. Although a bra isn't an absolute necessity in this period, you'll probably be more comfortable in one, at least if it fits well. If you leak milk and want to use breast pads, you'll definitely need a bra to hold them in place.

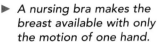 ▶ *A nursing bra makes the breast available with only the motion of one hand.*

A stretch bra that can be pulled out of the way may work fine if you're small-breasted, but otherwise you may prefer a nursing bra, with its removable cup flaps.

Pregnancy changes not only the size of the breasts but also the size of the rib cage. After you give birth, both measurements change again. If you buy a nursing bra in early pregnancy, it may not fit when milk productions begins. A better time to shop for nursing bras is during the last month of pregnancy. To be on the safe side, limit your purchase to two or three bras; you'll be more sure of the size and style that suits you after a week or so of nursing.

The salesperson in the maternity shop or department may be able to help you choose a bra that will fit well while you are nursing. If she doesn't know a lot about bras, though, you can figure out your size yourself by following these guidelines: While standing, wearing an unpadded bra and breathing normally, measure your chest just under your arms with a tape measure. Round up to an even number of inches; this number is your band size. Now measure around your body at the fullest part of your bust. As shown in the chart on the next page, the difference between the bust measurement and band size determines your cup size.

Since finding larger bra sizes can be difficult, you may have to use a mail-order supplier. To locate one, see Appendix A, page 242.

To check a bra for fit, fasten it on the outside row of hooks. Before raising the straps over your shoulders, bend forward, allowing your breasts to fill the cups. Now stand straight, and adjust the straps.

Difference Between Bust Measurement and Band Size	Cup Size
Up to 1-inch difference	A cup
1- to 2-inch difference	B cup
2- to 3-inch difference	C cup
3- to 4-inch difference	D cup
4- to 5-inch difference	DD or E cup
5- to 6-inch difference	F cup
6- to 7-inch difference	G cup
7- to 8-inch difference	H cup

Check the cup fit. When the flaps of a nursing bra are hooked at their highest points, the cups should have just a little extra room at the top for when milk production begins. If the cups are roomier than this, try a smaller cup size. If your breasts are overflowing at the top, outsides, or center, you need a larger cup size.

Next check the bottom band. While fastened on the outside row of hooks, the band should be snug; an inner row of hooks will allow you to tighten the band as your rib cage contracts after birth. Check to see that the band is level all around or slightly lower in the back. If the bra rides up in the back, the shoulder straps may be too tight. Otherwise, try a larger cup size.

Aside from a good fit, other valuable features of a bra for breast-feeding include all-cotton or microfiber cups to absorb moisture, non-elastic straps for better support, and front-flap fasteners that are manageable with one hand.

A word about underwire bras: Poorly fitted ones are associated with plugged milk ducts and breast infections. If you want to wear an underwire bra while nursing, it is very important to get one that fits properly. The bend of the wire must be wide enough to fall where there are no milk ducts—that is, well behind the breast tissue. If you have a lot of breast tissue below the armpits, as many women do, a soft-cup bra is definitely preferable. If you do use an underwire bra while nursing, alternate it with a soft-cup bra, and never wear the underwire bra during sleep.

You may also wish to purchase breast pads before delivery, to keep your bra and clothing dry during the early weeks of nursing (not all women leak, so you may want to start with just one pack). These pads come in two varieties, disposable and reusable. Whichever you select, be sure the pads do not contain plastic or waterproof liners, as these can contribute to nipple soreness. Some women prefer to use handkerchiefs or cut-up cloth diapers instead of commercial pads.

Sometimes mothers consider using plastic breast shells instead of pads to keep dry. The primary purpose of these shells is to improve nipple shape. When they are routinely worn in place of pads, milk may leak excessively.

Other purchases you may be considering

The arms of an adult are never a safe place for an infant or small child riding in an automobile. If you use a car, buy an infant restraining seat; every U.S. state now requires the use of one. Although all infant car seats sold today must meet federal safety standards, the seats vary considerably in both features and price. Look for latches you can operate easily; you may also prefer a washable cover. If you're considering a secondhand car seat, check its label to be sure it meets safety standards. Some communities and hospitals offer car seat rental and loan programs.

Don't pay extra for a car seat that also functions as a general-purpose infant carrier. In the past decade, plastic carriers, many of which double as car seats, have become one of the most harmful types of baby equipment. Parents use them both to carry their babies outside the home and to contain them within the home, whether the babies are awake or asleep. Some babies spend many hours each day in these carriers. The problem is that the carriers limit babies' movements and thereby delay their muscular and sensory-motor development. Babies need to spend most of their time in a horizontal position, in someone's arms or on a level surface. The constant upright position fails to stimulate the lower brain and delays physical coordination. A bouncer seat, bassinet, or blanket on the floor is a better place to leave your baby for extended periods. Or carry your baby in a pouch or sling, keeping your arms free for other things. Holding, rocking, and carrying your baby against your body will stimulate his physical and mental development while strengthening the loving bond between you.

You'll want to either buy diapers or arrange for diaper service for the first few weeks. Besides being ecologically safer than disposable diapers, cloth diapers are more economical as well, if you own or have access to a washer and dryer. Full diaper service is usually no more expensive than disposable diapers and is a luxury all new parents deserve.

A comfortable armchair can make positioning your newborn at the breast much easier and provide more support for you while nursing. Many couches are too deep to sit up straight on. Propping yourself against your headboard or sitting on the edge of the bed could make it hard to position your baby well and contribute to poor posture and muscle fatigue. An upholstered living-room, dining-room, or office chair with arms, or a wooden rocking chair, may make a great place for nursing your baby. If your breasts are large, a recliner may be most comfortable. Consider borrowing an appropriate chair or buying one secondhand if you can't afford to buy a new one.

Although ordinary bed pillows can work well in helping to position a baby for nursing, a variety of pillows are being marketed specifically for this purpose, and they are becoming very popular for the early weeks of nursing. If you'd like to try one of these pillows, choose one with flat surfaces rather than one that is crescent-shaped. Crescent-shaped pillows often create a gap between the pillow and the mother's body, and the baby tends to slip down in between.

Many mothers have found that a foot stool specially designed for nursing is very helpful in reducing the strain of holding the baby at the breast. The angled stool raises the mother's feet and legs, lifting her lap. This relaxes her abdomen and supports her lower back, preventing arm and shoulder strain. Nursing stools can be bought through some catalogs and from a major breast pump manufacturer (see Appendix A, page 247, for information on ordering them).

Some mothers buy breast pumps before delivery. Although a pump is not a necessity, you may at some time want to use one. Or you may prefer to learn the technique of manual expression, which is described on pages 175–176. If you decide to purchase a pump ahead of time, see pages 176–185 for a review of various popular models and information on obtaining them. Many mothers are disappointed with the pumps widely available in drugstores and baby shops.

Some mothers need a fully automatic electric breast pump in the first few days after delivery. Whether you buy another sort of pump or not, know where you can rent an electric pump should the need arise. If your baby isn't nursing well upon leaving the hospital or is at risk of underfeeding for another reason (see pages 39–40), you should go home with an electric pump. You can locate a rental station by calling the toll-free numbers in Appendix A, page 243.

PLANNING FOR THE FIRST WEEKS

During your first few weeks of motherhood, caring for the baby and yourself will take just about all of your time and energy. Most new mothers find they are often tired and have emotional highs and lows.

Planning ahead can make these important first weeks go much more smoothly for both you and your family.

If your partner can possibly manage to take time off from work, by all means encourage him to do so. Not only can he help in fixing meals, managing the household, and caring for any other children at home, but he also needs and deserves time to get to know the baby. And he can be a great source of support and encouragement while you are learning to breastfeed.

Other family members can also make these weeks easier, but invite them to stay with you only if you feel they will make a positive contribution and be supportive of your nursing.

Perhaps some of your friends in the area have already offered to help when the baby arrives. There are many things they can do, like fixing a meal, washing a load or two of laundry, running errands, minding any older children, or spending an hour or so straightening up your house.

It's also a good idea to stock up on groceries before the birth. Include foods that are easy to prepare and plenty of things to drink. You may also want to plan some simple menus or freeze some dinners ahead of time.

Your support system About half of American women who start out breastfeeding give up and begin bottle feeding within the first two months after birth. As said so well by Dana Raphael (1976), "The odds in our culture today are stacked heavily against successful breastfeeding, and the emotional price for failure is high." Mothers frequently give up breastfeeding in the learning stage because they have little information, guidance, and support.

When a nursing mother is encouraged and cared for by others, her motivation can carry her through almost any difficult situation. When she feels alone and unsupported, however, the nursing relationship seems to fall apart at the slightest provocation.

As enthusiastic as you may feel now, you probably have difficulty imagining that during the early weeks you may sometimes doubt your ability to nurse. In fact, many new mothers experience periods of anxiety while they are learning to breastfeed. If you are lucky you can turn to your own mother for advice and reassurance about nursing. Many of our mothers, however, nursed us only a few weeks, if at all. You may hear from today's grandmothers that "no one nursed back then," "the doctor said the bottle was easier," "I just didn't make enough milk," or "the doctor said my milk wasn't rich enough."

Comments such as these reflect an era when women received little encouragement and support in their efforts to nurse, especially from their male doctors. Consider for a moment the idea of giving birth all alone. Awful, right? It is probably important to you that someone you love and trust will be with you, encouraging you each step of the way. During your early weeks of breastfeeding you need the same kind of support—the presence of someone who provides reassurance, guidance, and encouragement.

You may be fortunate enough to have friends who have nursed—or are nursing—their babies, and a partner who believes with you that breastfeeding is healthy and natural. Even so, you may discover in time that not everyone in your life shares your feelings about breastfeeding. In fact, many people feel indifferent, and some downright opposed, to this way of feeding and nurturing a baby. Your partner, mother, or best friend may not be entirely enthusiastic about your decision. Some people may even try to discourage you along the way. Perhaps they feel a bit threatened, fearful, or even jealous of the intimate relationship you will be establishing with the baby. The sad fact of the matter is that despite the renewed enthusiasm of young women today toward breastfeeding, many new mothers still get too little support—from family, friends, health professionals, and society in general.

Develop a support system for yourself ahead of time. Let your partner and other family members know how much breastfeeding means to you and how important they will be to your success. If they have concerns or fears about nursing, find out what they are and provide them with the information they need to correct any misconceptions. If you have older children, talk with them about nursing so they know what to expect.

Be sure to identify sources of guidance. Perhaps you are close to women who have successfully nursed their babies. Many WIC (Women, Infants, and Children Supplemental Nutrition) programs provide breastfeeding support and guidance (see page 241 for more information about WIC). Take time to find the names of lactation professionals in your community. Your childbirth educator, your maternity unit, or your obstetrician's or pediatrician's nurse may know of some, and WIC programs sometimes have lactation professionals on staff. Two breast pump companies, Medela and Ameda, have geographically arranged lists of lactation professionals. When you have gathered these supports, you will have stacked the odds in your favor.

2 OFF TO A GOOD START: THE FIRST WEEK

In the Beginning
Ensuring Your Milk Supply
The First Week of Nursing

You might expect that after the work of labor and birth a mother and her newborn infant would be too exhausted to greet each other. But no matter how fatigued birth may have left her, the mother usually brightens with renewed energy to explore her baby. Some mothers seem to meet their infants for the first time with puzzlement, as if searching for some sign of familiarity. Others react as if they have always known this tiny being and are overjoyed to meet him at long last.

After several minutes of adjustment to breathing, the temperature change, and lights and sounds, the infant likewise becomes alert, opening his eyes and moving his mouth. Soon he is actively rooting about. With his fists to his mouth, or perhaps his lips against the blanket or his father's arm, he seeks out the comfort of the breast.

IN THE BEGINNING

Throughout the first two hours after birth, the infant is usually alert and eager to suck. At this time he is most ready for his first nursing.

Colostrum

It is not unusual to hear a first-time mother tell a nurse, "I don't think I have anything yet to feed the baby." Although small in amount, colostrum is available in the breast in quantities close to the stomach capacity of the newborn. This "liquid gold," which is often yellow, but may be clear, resembles blood more than milk in that it contains protective white blood cells capable of attacking harmful bacteria. Colostrum also acts to "seal" the inside of the baby's intestines, preventing the invasion of bacteria, and provides the baby with high levels of antibodies from the mother. Not only does colostrum thus offer protection from sickness, but it is the ideal food for the newborn's first few days of life. It is high in protein and low in sugar and fat, making it easy to digest. Colostrum is also beneficial in stimulating the baby's early bowel movements. The black, tarry stool, called meconium, contains bilirubin, the substance that causes newborn jaundice. Colostrum in frequent doses helps eliminate bilirubin from the body and may lessen the incidence and severity of jaundice.

In the hospital this first nursing may take place in the delivery room, the birthing room, or the recovery area. With minimal assistance from your nurse or partner, the baby will probably latch on eagerly to the breast and suck. He will be more willing if he is unbundled; snuggled within your arm and next to your body, he is unlikely to get too cold (unless perhaps the room is air-conditioned). The purple color of his hands and feet is normal; it is caused by changes in blood circulation that take place at delivery. If you or the nurse is concerned about the cold, place a blanket over the baby after he has begun to nurse.

Many specialists believe that when the first nursing is delayed much beyond the first two hours, the infant may be somewhat reluctant to take the breast thereafter. Most babies fall asleep about two hours after birth, and become more difficult to rouse over the next few hours. Nursing without delay also boosts the confidence of the mother, and stimulates the action of hormones that cause the uterus to contract and remain firm after delivery. These contractions may help speed delivery of the placenta and minimize blood loss afterward (breastfeeding alone is insufficient, however, in the case of postpartum hemorrhage, when prompt intervention by the medical staff is essential). During the first few days after birth, some mothers feel these contractions, or "afterpains," while nursing. Mothers who have had other children may be especially uncomfortable with afterpains.

Should you not have the opportunity to nurse right after delivery, or if you can't persuade your baby to take the breast, don't get discouraged. Many mothers have established successful nursing hours or days after giving birth.

Just the breast

When you have finished your first nursing in the hospital, let the nurses know (if you have not done so previously) that you prefer your baby be given no supplementary bottles of water or formula and no pacifiers. Water or formula is unnecessary, and artificial nipples may confuse your baby while he is learning to breastfeed.

Newborns do not normally require any fluids other than colostrum (the exception is the baby who has low blood sugar—because her mother is diabetic, her birth weight was low, or she underwent unusual stress during labor or delivery). Supplemental feedings, moreover, can be harmful: they may cause the baby to lose interest in the breast and to nurse less frequently than needed. This is because bottle nipples may (1) lessen the baby's instinctive efforts to open her mouth wide, (2) condition her to wait to suck until she feels the firm bottle nipple in her mouth, and (3) encourage her to push her tongue forward—the opposite of what she needs to do while nursing. The baby who has sucked on bottle nipples may also become frustrated while nursing, since milk does not flow as rapidly from the breast as it does from the bottle.

Giving newborns large amounts of water is dangerous. Because young babies can't excrete water quickly, large amounts can lower sodium levels in their bodies, causing complications that include low body temperature and seizures.

A newborn trained to take a pacifier may fail to recognize her mother's soft, short nipple, and therefore have trouble latching on to the breast. Introducing a pacifier now could lead to later problems, too. Recent studies associate the use of pacifiers with early weaning, and older babies who use pacifiers are more likely than others to have frequent ear infections.

Some hospitals now have policies against giving bottles and pacifiers to nursing newborns, but not all do. To be sure all the nurses know of your preference, ask them to place a sign on the baby's crib like this one:

To all my nurses:
While I'm here and learning to breastfeed, PLEASE, NO BOTTLES OR PACIFIERS. My mom will be happy to nurse me whenever I fuss.

Thanks!!
Baby Reynolds

Time at the breast

Many doctors and nurses tell mothers that to prevent sore nipples they should limit their nursing time during the first several days. Probably nothing else about breastfeeding is as poorly understood as the causes of sore nipples. It may be explained that keeping feedings short will prevent soreness and will help "toughen" the nipples. Actually, sore nipples usually result from improper positioning of the baby on the breast, not from long nursings. Another myth often heard by new mothers is that the breast "empties" in a prescribed number of minutes. Most newborns require 10 to 45 minutes to complete a feeding. As long as your positioning is correct and nursing is comfortable, there is no need to restrict your nursing time. Besides being unnecessary, limiting nursing time may frustrate the baby and lead to increased engorgement when milk production begins.

Positioning at the breast

A baby is correctly positioned at the breast when he has latched on to it with a wide-open mouth, so that his lower gum is well below the base of the nipple on the areola, the dark area around the nipples. In this position he will compress the sinuses located beneath the areola to draw out milk. If he instead latches on to the nipple only and starts "chewing," the nipple will probably become sore and cracked, and perhaps even bleed. The baby will also be unable to compress the sinuses beneath the areola and may therefore get too little milk.

Probably the most important skill for you to master, initially, is that of getting the baby on the breast correctly. Some mothers can do this easily, but many need practice.

The "cradle hold," or "cuddle hold," in which the baby's head is held in the crook of the mother's arm, is considered the classic breastfeeding position. I have come to believe that for most new mothers

▶ *An infant correctly positioned while nursing.*

▶ *It's hard to control a newborn's
head using the cradle hold.*

and babies this position is neither the easiest nor the most effective
for getting a baby well latched on to the breast. In the first few weeks
after birth, a baby hasn't developed enough muscular coordination of
the head and neck to easily latch on without help; she needs a good
deal of direction from her mother. But it is difficult to direct a newborn's head accurately with the inside of one's forearm. Although
most mothers sooner or later begin using the cradle hold for most of
their daytime nursings, in the early days of breastfeeding the cross-
over and football holds are generally more useful.

The cross-over hold. Take time to position yourself comfortably. If
you are nursing in a hospital bed, sit up as straight as possible with a
pillow behind you. As soon as you are able, sit in a chair with arms
(most couches are too deep). Unwrap your baby; this will encourage
his interest in latching on and make it easier for you to check his position. Place one or two pillows on your lap so that the baby is at the
level of your breast. Lay him on his side with his chest and abdomen
against your body.

Instead of placing the baby's head in the bend of your elbow as in
the cradle hold, hold him with the opposite arm, so that your hand
rests between his shoulder blades and supports the back of his neck
and head. Place your thumb behind and below one ear and your
other fingers behind and below the other ear. Tip his head back
slightly so that, when you pull him onto the breast, his chin will reach
it first. Now shift the baby, if necessary, so that his nose—not his
mouth—is right in front of your nipple. In this position he is most
likely to latch on with his lower jaw well below the base of the nipple.

If you're starting on the left breast, hold it with your left hand so
that your thumb is positioned at the margin of the areola, about 1½
inches from the nipple, at the spot where the baby's nose will touch
the breast (or at about two o'clock, if you imagine a clock face

▲ *Cross-over hold*

▲ *Hand position for the cross-over hold*

printed on your breast). Place your index finger the same distance from the nipple at the spot where the baby's chin will touch the breast (or at about eight o'clock). Gently compress the breast to match the shape of your baby's open mouth.

Before you bring the baby onto the breast, you must stimulate him to "root." Touch the baby just under the nose with your nipple, and wait until he opens his mouth wide. When his lower jaw is dropped all the way down, quickly bring his shoulders and head together to the breast. With his head tipped slightly back, his chin

▲ *Just before latch-on: Tip the baby's head back a bit, and aim your nipple at his upper lip.*

▲ *Just before latch-on, from your point of view*

should reach the breast first. Don't lean into the baby. Keep the areola compressed until he begins sucking. You'll know that he is well latched on if his lips are far apart and flared, if he has more of the bottom of the areola in his mouth than the top, and if you feel comfortable.

You may need to repeat this process several times before the baby latches on correctly. Common mistakes include lining up the baby's mouth rather than the nose with the nipple, pulling the baby on before his mouth is wide open, not pulling him on quick enough or far enough, and letting go of the breast before he is well latched on.

Once the baby is actively nursing, you'll probably need to support the breast for him, by gently pressing your fingers against the underside. If your breasts are small, though, you may be able to let go of the breast or even switch arms and continue nursing using the cradle hold.

Football hold. The football hold is a great position to use when—

- You have had a cesarean birth and want to avoid placing the baby against your abdomen.
- You need more visibility in getting the baby to latch on.
- Your breasts are large.
- You are nursing a small baby, especially if he is premature.
- You are nursing twins.

Sit in a comfortable armchair with a pillow at your side to help support your arm and lift the baby. Support the baby in a semisitting position facing you, with her bottom at the back of the chair. Your

▲ *Football hold*

▲ *Hand position for the football hold*

arm closest to your baby should support her back, with your hand holding her neck and head. Place your thumb behind and below one ear and your other fingers behind the other ear. Position the baby with her head just below the breast and her nose in front of the nipple. This way she'll latch on to the areola with her lower jaw well below the base of the nipple.

Support your breast with your free hand so that your thumb is about $1\frac{1}{2}$ inches above the nipple, at twelve o'clock, and your index finger is the same distance below the nipple, at six o'clock. Compress the areola with your thumb and index finger so that your hand forms a C-shape. This will more closely match your breast to the shape of your baby's mouth, so she can take in more of the breast. As with the cross-over hold, stimulate the baby to open her mouth wide, and bring her up onto the breast.

Side-lying position. The side-lying position is an especially good choice for nursing when—

- You must be flat after a cesarean birth.
- You are uncomfortable sitting up.
- You need help from someone else to get the baby latched on.
- The baby is sleepy and reluctant to begin nursing or stay awake very long.
- You are nursing during the night.

▲ *Side-lying position*

You and your baby lie on your sides, tummy to tummy, as with the cuddle hold. Place your fingers beneath the breast and lift upward, then pull the baby in close after he roots with a wide open mouth.

The side-lying position becomes much easier after four to six weeks, when the baby has better head control and can come onto the breast without much assistance.

| **Ending the feeding** | Waiting until your baby lets go of the nipple is the ideal way to end a feeding. If the baby does |

not come off the breast by himself after 20 to 25 minutes on a side, and you want to switch breasts or rest awhile, you can take him off by first breaking the suction. Even if he is not actively sucking, his hold on the nipple is tremendously strong. To release the suction, insert your finger into the corner of his mouth, pushing your finger between his gums until you hear or feel the release. You can also try placing your finger on the corner of the baby's mouth and pulling the skin gently towards his ear.

After taking the baby off the breast, leave your bra flaps down so that the air can dry your nipples. Air drying helps to maintain healthy nipples.

| **After a cesarean birth** | Whether or not your cesarean is planned, your milk will come in just as if you had delivered vaginally, and you can breastfeed your baby. |

Because you will be recovering from surgery, you will face some discomfort and possibly some difficulty maneuvering the baby to your breast. If you are expecting a cesarean, you may want to ask to share a hospital room with another woman who has had one. Some hospitals make such arrangements routinely.

If you are awake for your delivery, let the staff and the baby's physician know you wish to nurse as soon as possible. As long as the baby is not having any difficulties, there is no reason to delay nursing. If you can't sit up, you can nurse in the side-lying position with some help from your partner or the nurse.

If you are not fully conscious during the delivery, or if the baby is kept in the nursery by the doctor's orders, you can still begin nursing after your initial separation. Medication for pain is important for your comfort during the first few days; it will not hurt the baby. If you take the medication right after you nurse, moreover, only a minimal amount will be in your milk at the next feeding. After a couple of days you may want to keep the baby in the room with you.

Remember to ask for help whenever you need it. Sometimes the staff may forget you gave birth by cesarean section.

You may prefer to nurse at first in the side-lying position. Leave the side rails of the bed up so that turning will be easier. A pillow behind your back and one between your legs may be helpful. When you begin sitting up to nurse, a pillow on your lap will make you more comfortable. The football hold works well while sitting if you want to keep the baby off your abdomen.

ENSURING YOUR MILK SUPPLY

Frequent nursing

Your baby should be nursing often, at least eight times in 24 hours. Until your milk comes in your baby needs frequent feedings of colostrum. After your milk comes in, about 72 hours after the birth, a good feeding every few hours will help ensure a plentiful milk supply.

During the first few days after birth, many babies are sleepy. If your newborn has not nursed after three hours (counted from the start of the last feeding), unwrap her from her blankets, rub her back, and talk to her. She will probably then become interested in nursing.

In the hospital, keeping the baby with you in your room helps ensure frequent nursing. If you are not rooming-in with your baby, ask the nurses to bring her to you at least every three hours (more often if she fusses), including whenever she wakens in the night.

Encourage the baby to have a good feeding each time you nurse her. Until your milk is in, you can probably persuade her to take both breasts at each feeding. Listen for the sound of your baby swallowing; when you hear it you will know that she is taking colostrum or milk. When your baby has released the nipple, or when you have nursed her for 20 to 25 minutes and she is no longer swallowing, burp her. Hold her up over your shoulder and pat her back, or sit her upright, bent slightly forward with your hand supporting her lower jaw, and firmly pat her lower back. After burping, she will probably regain interest in nursing and take the second breast. If she doesn't burp within a few minutes, just switch sides. If she refuses to nurse on the second breast or nurses only a short time, be sure to start her on that side at the next feeding.

The first days of milk production are the critical period for determining whether a mother ends up with a generous milk supply or an inadequate one. If little milk is removed from the breast, the resulting pressure causes the breast to slow down production. If no milk is

▶ *You can burp the baby by sitting her up, one hand under her jaw. Firmly pat her lower back with the other hand.*

removed, milk production stops entirely. (This is how women who don't nurse stop producing milk.) So ensuring a good milk supply depends on having a vigorous nursing baby (or an effective breast pump) that drains at least one breast every few hours around the clock.

Avoiding supplements

Another way to help ensure your milk supply is to avoid supplemental feedings. Some babies become very confused when a bottle nipple is introduced during the first few days (see "Just the Breast," page 29). Glucose (sugar) water offers few calories and may discourage the baby's interest in nursing. Also, babies fed glucose water more frequently develop jaundice in the first few days after birth. After taking formula, a baby frequently will not want to nurse for four hours or longer, since formula takes longer to digest than breast milk. The decrease in breast stimulation may decrease milk production.

Putting your fears to rest

In the early days of nursing, you may be very surprised at how often your baby wants to nurse. Like many newborns, yours may seem fussy and hungry much of the time. This may make you wonder if you have enough milk, and if you should pump your milk and feed it by bottle to see how much the baby is getting. Well-meaning friends and family members may even suggest you supplement your milk with formula.

Most newborns want to nurse eight to twelve times in each 24-hour period after the first day or two post partum. This frequent nursing is normal; it seldom reflects a poor milk supply and it never reflects "weak milk." Unless you or your baby falls into one of the categories described under "Babies Who May Not Get Enough" (page 39), your baby is probably getting plenty of milk.

Without introducing a bottle, though, how can you know your baby is getting enough? You can look for these signs of adequate milk intake:

- *Your milk has come in by the third or fourth day post partum.* When milk production begins, the breasts become firmer and heavier. The firmness may be less apparent with large breasts, but the breasts should still feel heavier.

- *Your baby is nursing at least eight times in a 24-hour period.* This means your baby is nursing every two to three hours (measured from the start of one feeding to the start of the next) during the day, with a sleep stretch of up to five hours at night. If your baby isn't nursing this often, you may have to wake her for feedings.

- *Your baby is nursing 10 to 45 minutes at each feeding and seems content after feedings.* Babies vary in the length of time they nurse, but they typically need 10 to 45 minutes to complete a feeding. Although babies don't always fall asleep after nursing, they should usually seem satisfied after feedings.

- *Your baby has several periods of swallowing during each feeding.* When babies are getting milk, they take long, drawing sucks and can be heard swallowing or gulping. (When they are not swallowing milk, they take short, choppy sucks.) These long, drawing sucks usually occur in burst of five to ten continuous sucks followed by a pause. Babies who are taking enough milk usually have several bursts of continuous sucking and swallowing during a feeding.

- *Your breasts feel softer or lighter after the baby has nursed.* You should be able to feel a difference in fullness or heaviness in your breasts before and after your baby has fed.

- *Your baby is having bowel movements every day, and by the fifth day they have turned yellow.* This is the clearest sign that a baby is getting enough colostrum, first, and, later, breast milk. Most newborns have at least three bowel movements each day during the first month. Only after the first month is it normal for breastfed babies to go several days without a bowel movement.

- *Your baby is wetting more diapers by the fifth day after birth.* Before your milk comes in, your baby will urinate infrequently, but by the fifth day you should notice more frequent and wetter diapers. Be aware that the more absorbent disposable diapers can make wetness difficult to detect.

If not all of the points just listed hold true for you and your baby, you should have him weighed and examined. In the first four to five days after birth, a baby loses weight. After the fifth day, a baby should gain an ounce every day. An initial loss of 10 percent or more of a baby's birth weight suggests the baby is underfed (see the chart in Appendix B, page 251). Even if your baby has lost less than 10 percent of his birth weight, have him weighed again in a couple of days to see if he has started gaining an ounce per day.

Babies who may not get enough

Some mothers and babies at risk for underfeeding can be identified even before the milk comes in. This group includes—

- babies who are born three weeks or more before the due date;
- babies who weigh less than six pounds at birth;
- babies who may have poor muscle tone, such as those with Down syndrome;
- babies who have unusual conformations in their mouths, such as a short frenulum (the string of tissue on the underside of the tongue) near the tongue's tip, a high palate, or a cleft lip or palate;
- mothers with large nipples (as large or larger in diameter than a quarter); and
- babies who aren't yet latching on or sustaining sucking 24 hours after birth.

If you or your baby falls into one of these risk groups, a few days of sluggish nursing and limited milk removal could have a devastating effect on your milk production. Consider renting a fully automatic electric breast pump, which may be more reliable than your baby in stimulating continued milk production. Starting on the third day after birth, pump for 5 minutes on each breast right after each daytime and evening nursing. If your baby isn't able to latch on or clearly isn't sucking effectively, start pumping earlier than the third day, and pump each breast for 10 to 15 minutes. This "insurance pumping" should assure that you'll have an abundant milk supply even if your baby's sucking is on the sluggish side. You can freeze the pumped milk for later use.

Watch your baby closely for the reassuring signs of adequate milk intake listed on pages 38–39. The baby should be weighed at 10 to 12 days of age, or sooner if you suspect that he may not be taking enough milk. If he has regained his birth weight, you can gradually stop pumping over a few days (before returning the pump, though, make sure the baby has gained an ounce a day since the last weighing). But if he is still below his birth weight at 10 to 12 days of age, supplement nursings with the pumped milk (see "Treatment Measures for Underfeeding," page 77).

Other babies who may not get enough milk are those whose mothers—

- have had previous breast surgery involving an incision around the nipple or areola, such as in some breast augmentation or reduction procedures (see "Nursing after Breast Surgery," page 86); or

- have widely spaced breasts that are rather long and thin, that did not get larger in pregnancy, and that may differ markedly from each other in size (see page 85).

In the latter case, such breasts are called hypoplastic. On the third day after birth, when the breasts normally fill with milk, hypoplastic breasts may remain soft. Because of a congenital abnormality, they contain insufficient glandular tissue, and so are unable to produce very much milk.

If you have had breast surgery that may affect your ability to produce milk, or if you suspect you may have insufficient glandular tissue, observe your baby closely for signs of low milk intake. Weigh her at three to four days of age and every couple of days thereafter until she is clearly gaining an ounce a day. If she loses 10 percent or more of her birth weight or does not gain an ounce a day after five days of age, she needs your pumped breast milk or formula as a supplement. See "Underfeeding and Weight Loss," page 76.

THE FIRST WEEK OF NURSING

Although most babies are alert and eager to nurse during the first two hours after birth, during the next few days they may sleep much of the time. The average baby, after the first couple of days, begins to wake up to nurse about every one to three hours. At night, he will sleep from one to five hours at a stretch. If your baby is not waking on his own to nurse at least eight times in each 24-hour period, including at least once in the night, awaken him for feedings.

The typical length of a feeding varies greatly from baby to baby.

A baby who is "all business"—who sucks and swallows with few pauses—may complete a feeding in as little as ten minutes. At the other extreme is the "dawdler," who sucks and swallows five or six times and then pauses. This pattern of frequent pausing may extend a feeding up to 45 minutes. Most babies' feedings fall between these extremes; the average is about 20 to 30 minutes. Although your baby may not fall asleep after feeding, he should seem content.

While the baby nurses, you should hear a lot of swallowing. Some babies gulp noisily, whereas others are more quiet. When babies are getting milk they take long, drawing sucks and can be heard swallowing or gulping. (They take short, choppy sucks when they are not swallowing milk.) These long, drawing sucks usually occur in bursts, that is, five to ten continuous sucks followed by a pause. Babies who are taking enough milk usually have several bursts of continuous sucking and swallowing during a feeding.

You should not hear clicking noises while your baby nurses. Clicking usually means that the baby is not sucking adequately and therefore may not be receiving enough milk. The baby should have such a strong hold on the breast that the nipple does not easily slip from his mouth when you pull him slightly away. His cheeks should remain smooth with each suck; dimples on the cheek while nursing are a sign of inadequate suction and faulty sucking (see "Sucking Problems," page 73, if your baby's cheeks are dimpling).

During the first day after birth, babies sometimes spit up mucus they have swallowed during delivery. Occasionally a baby will gag on this mucus. After the first 24 hours, this is usually no longer a problem.

Some babies also spit up colostrum or milk. The amounts are usually smaller than they seem, though you may wonder if your baby is keeping anything down. Spitting up a teaspoon or two after feedings is normal for some babies in the first week.

Babies also get hiccoughs, often after a feeding. If the baby starts hiccoughing after nursing at the first breast, it may be difficult to interest him in the other. You don't need to give him water or anything else. The hiccoughs are painless for him; just wait until they go away.

The baby's first stools, called meconium, are black and sticky. Stooling every day and having yellow stools by the fifth day usually indicates an adequate intake of colostrum, first, and then breast milk. This is one of the surest signs that a newborn is getting enough to eat. Most newborns have at least three bowel movements each day during the first month. Only after the first month is it normal for breastfed babies to go several days without having a bowel movement.

The yellow stools are soft, loose, or watery, and sometimes they look seedy. Babies normally strain and grunt when passing their stools—this does not mean they are constipated.

Wet diapers are usually infrequent in the first few days, but they should be more frequent and wetter by the fifth day. Eight or more diapers wet with pale urine each day, along with daily yellow stools, are usually a sign of sufficient milk intake. (This rule may not hold true if the baby is receiving water supplements.)

All newborns lose weight after birth. Expect your baby to lose about 5 to 9 percent of his birth weight. He should begin gaining weight by the fifth day, about an ounce a day.

Caring for your breasts

Your daily bath or shower is sufficient for cleaning your breasts. Avoid getting soap or shampoo on the nipple and areola; it tends to counteract the naturally occurring oils that cleanse this area. Antiseptic applications to the nipples are also unnecessary, but do take care to wash your hands before nursing.

You will probably want to wear a nursing bra for convenience and comfort, especially after your milk comes in. Again, bras with cotton or microfiber rather than synthetic cups allow for better air circulation to the nipples.

If the baby does not come off the breast by herself when the nursing session is over, take care to release the suction with your finger. Leave your breasts exposed to the air for five or ten minutes before covering up. Air drying is soothing to the nipples.

During the past decade nursing mothers have been discouraged from using nipple creams, since some women develop sore nipples in reaction to preparations containing lanolin, vitamin E, or cocoa butter. Also, lanolin preparations were discovered to be contaminated with pesticide residues. Recently, however, a purified form of lanolin has been developed: it is nonallergenic and pesticide-free. Modified lanolin will not prevent nipple soreness, but it is very soothing to tender nipples and may promote healing. See Appendix A, page 247, for ordering information.

For those women who leak milk, nursing pads are usually necessary during this time to prevent wet or spotted clothing. You can buy the pads in two varieties: reusable, washable types, and disposable types. (Remember: if you prefer disposable pads, stay away from those with plastic liners because they keep the nipple wet and may aggravate soreness.)

If you are using plastic breast shells to improve the shape of your nipples, you may find during the first few weeks that they cause your milk to leak excessively and keep your nipples damp. You might try placing the shells in your bra just 20 to 30 minutes before the feeding (milk collected this way must be discarded). Don't routinely use breast shells in place of nursing pads; this would probably cause more leakage. Breast shells should be washed after each nursing in hot soapy water and rinsed thoroughly.

When your milk comes in
Milk production generally begins on the second or third day post partum, but occasionally not until the fourth day. At first the milk will be mixed with colostrum, and so will be pale orange in color. After a few days the milk will become whiter. This mature milk will look more watery than cow's milk; it may resemble skim milk. If your milk hasn't come in by the fourth day after birth, see "Late Onset of Milk Production," page 49.

Most women notice that their breasts become larger, fuller, and more tender as the milk comes in. Large-breasted women may notice only a change in heaviness. This change, known as engorgement, is caused by increased blood flow to the breasts as well as beginning milk production. Fullness may be more apparent if your breasts are normally small or medium-sized. They may feel lumpy, and the lumpiness may extend all the way to your armpits, since milk glands are also located there. After nursing, your breasts should feel softer or lighter.

Engorgement normally lasts 24 to 48 hours. During this time a nursing bra will provide support and comfort. Frequent nursing, at least every two to three hours, is the best treatment. Heat treatments such as warm showers, hot packs, and heating pads may worsen the swelling. You may get relief, though, from gently massaging the breast while the baby is nursing. This will encourage more milk to let down. It is important to pay careful attention to the way the baby latches on while the breast is engorged. When latch-on is incorrect, because the baby isn't positioned well or the areola is overly full, soreness often follows. If the areola is hard, you can express some milk, by hand or with a pump. (For further advice on managing engorgement, see page 48.)

When you put your baby to breast you may feel any of these normal sensations: warmth, relaxation, sleepiness, thirst, and even hunger.

It is normal for milk to leak from the breasts. When the baby nurses at one breast, milk may drip from the other. This leaking may continue for several weeks, or it may never happen at all.

From hospital to home At the time of discharge it is customary in many hospitals to give new mothers an array of sample products that manufacturers would like them to try. It may appear that the staff endorses these products; this is not necessarily so. One of these gifts is usually a package of formula, sometimes called a "breastfeeding kit." The "kit" contains formula, bottle nipples, and a pamphlet on breastfeeding. These pamphlets sometimes contain misleading information about nursing. Since you have chosen to breastfeed, it is best to leave the kit behind. You won't be needing it.

What are well worth taking home, however, are the names and telephone numbers of people who have a good reputation for helping nursing mothers and infants. Ask any nurse who has been encouraging or helpful with your early breastfeeding for this information. She may know of volunteers in La Leche League or the Nursing Mothers Counsel, or lactation professionals in your community.

At home. As any experienced nursing mother can tell you, the first few days at home with a baby are exhausting and, at times, emotional. These days are best spent caring only for yourself and the baby. Besides recovering from the birth, you are doing the important work of getting to know your baby and learning to breastfeed. Rest and a quiet, pleasant environment are important in preventing anxiety and "baby blues." Try to eat well, but don't worry if your appetite has lessened; this can be normal during the first couple of weeks after delivery. Ideally, you should spend the first several days nursing and resting with the baby, while a supportive partner or helper (or both) manages your home, meals, and callers.

If you have another child or children, you'll want help with them, too. Otherwise you may find yourself feeling suddenly, unexpectedly impatient or irritable with a beloved older child. When my second child was born, I found myself wishing someone could take away my nine-year-old for a while. Such feelings may arise from a natural protective urge that allows a mother to focus her total attention on the vulnerable newborn; shifting hormones and lack of sleep may contribute, too. Other species also defend their babies aggressively. For instance, picking up the new babies of a household pet may make the new mama growl, though in a few weeks she may not care at all when someone handles them.

In women, as in cats and dogs, such feelings usually lessen over time. In the meantime, they present a fine opportunity for your older child to strengthen a relationship with Dad, Grandma or Grandpa, or another adult. This is also a great chance for your older child to learn patience and responsibility. You can encourage him to accept the big-kid role by saying outright that "the baby comes first." Your child may feel proud to help by fetching a diaper or glass of water, and he may later be able to apply the baby-comes-first principle with other helpless creatures, such as pets.

It is not uncommon for things to suddenly "fall apart" shortly after a new mother comes home from the hospital. Suddenly responsible for a new baby, you may feel shaky at times and your confidence may vanish. The dramatic hormonal shift that begins immediately after birth may also affect your emotional state for a short time. You may find yourself exhausted and upset—especially if you've been taking responsibility for more than the baby and yourself.

Many new mothers have times when they feel that nursing "isn't working" and think about giving it up. Combined with the mood swings that follow birth, fears that the baby may not be getting enough milk, struggles with getting the baby to latch on, or problems like sore nipples can be overwhelming. Despite tearful moments, rest assured that most early nursing difficulties can be overcome with patience and help. Don't hesitate to track down assistance. Just a phone conversation with a knowledgeable person may be enough to get you and your baby back on track.

The postpartum period is a time of physical and emotional adjustment. As with most of life's great transitions, this one is usually accompanied by some turmoil. It will take several weeks, and most of your time and energy, to get to know your baby and learn how to care for her. So don't do more than you must, and accept offers for help. Adjusting to motherhood is always easier when you are supported and cared for by others.

THE FIRST WEEK

CONCERNS ABOUT YOURSELF

Engorged Breasts
Late Onset of Milk Production
Sore Nipples
Breast Pain
Leaking Milk
Let-down Difficulty
Milk Appearance
Difficult Latch-on: Flat,
    Dimpled, or Inverted Nipples
Fatigue and Depression

CONCERNS ABOUT THE BABY

Sleepy Baby
Bowel Movements
Jaundice
Difficult Latch-on:
    Refusal to Nurse
Sucking Problems
Fussiness and Excessive
    Night Waking
Underfeeding and
    Weight Loss

CONCERNS ABOUT YOURSELF

Engorged breasts

At two or three days post partum the breasts usually become engorged, or temporarily swollen. This is caused by the increased flow of blood to the breasts and the start of milk production. For some women the breasts become only slightly full, but for others they feel very swollen, tender, throbbing, and lumpy. Sometimes the swelling extends all the way to the armpit. Engorgement may cause the nipple to flatten, making it difficult for the baby to latch on. The problem usually lessens within 24 to 48 hours, but the swelling and discomfort may worsen if nursing is too brief or infrequent or if the baby sucks ineffectively. If engorgement is unrelieved by nursing or pumping, milk production declines and ultimately stops altogether.

Although many health-care providers recommend applying direct heat (warm washcloths, heating pads, hot water bottles, or hot showers) to engorged breasts, this may actually aggravate engorgement.

Treatment Measures for Engorged Breasts

1. Wear a supportive nursing bra, even during the night. Be sure your bra is not too tight.
2. Nurse frequently, every one to three hours. This may mean waking the baby (see "Sleepy Baby," page 63).
3. Avoid having the baby latch on when the areola is very firm. To reduce the possibility of damage to your nipples, manually express or pump milk until the areola softens. Wearing plastic breast shells for half an hour before nursing also helps to soften the areola.
4. Encourage the baby to nurse at least 10 minutes or longer at each breast. It is preferable to nurse on just one side until the breast is soft, even if the baby then goes to sleep, than to limit the baby's nursing time on the first side so you can nurse from both sides in one feeding.
5. Gently massage the breast at which the baby is nursing. This will encourage the milk to flow and will help relieve some of the tightness and discomfort you feel.
6. To soothe the pain and help relieve swelling, apply a cold pack to the breast for a short period *after* nursing. You can use ice in a plastic bag, or, better, soak a disposable diaper in water, shape it, and then freeze it. Lay a thin cloth over your breast before applying the cold diaper.

◄ *The breasts may grow astonishingly big and hard as milk production begins.*

7. If you need to, take acetaminophen tablets (such as Tylenol), ibuprofen (such as Advil or Motrin), or another mild pain reliever.

8. If 48 hours after your milk has come in you still find yourself overly full right after nursing, use a pump to drain both breasts as completely as possible. In this first week, habitual pumping along with nursing is generally discouraged, as it can lead to more engorgement and chronic overproduction. But pumping after nursing once every 24 hours or so should relieve your engorgement, not prolong it.

9. If the baby is not nursing well enough to soften at least one breast every few hours, use an electric breast pump as necessary. Unrelieved engorgement causes milk production to stop.

Late onset of milk production

Within 72 hours after birth, the production of mature milk normally begins. The breasts typically feel heavier and fuller, although large-breasted women may notice little change.

Occasionally milk production is delayed beyond 72 hours; sometimes it begins only days later. In the meantime, the breasts remain soft, and the baby sucks but gets little milk. In these circumstances, some babies seem sleepy and content, but most act hungry and dissatisfied. They have infrequent bowel movements and lose more weight than normally expected.

I suspect that events during labor and birth may influence the onset of milk production. Overhydration with intravenous fluids during a long or induced labor, or after a postpartum hemorrhage, may perhaps cause a delay in mature milk production.

If your milk is late in coming in, you may need to supplement with formula until it does. But you should continue to nurse frequently in the meantime.

Treatment Measures for Late Onset of Milk Production

1. If after 72 hours post partum you suspect that your milk is not in, have your baby weighed. If he has lost less than 10 percent of his birth weight (see the chart in Appendix B, page 251), continue to nurse frequently, every one to three hours, and monitor his weight daily.

2. If the baby has lost 10 percent or more of his birth weight, use an electric breast pump after each nursing. Feed your baby the colostrum you collect and any necessary formula (see Appendix B, page 251, to determine how much your baby needs).

3. When your milk comes in, refer to "Underfeeding and Weight Loss," page 76, to estimate your production and wean your baby off formula and pumped milk.

Sore nipples

There is no doubt about it: sore nipples can make a trial of what ought to be a joyous experience. For a few days after giving birth, you may feel slight tenderness during the first minute of nursing, when the baby latches on and the nipple stretches into her mouth. Such tenderness is normal at this time. (See "General Comfort Measures for Sore Nipples," page 51.)

If your nipples become really sore, however, they are probably damaged or irritated and require treatment beyond simple comfort measures. It is important for you to identify the cause of the problem so that you can help your nipples heal. At any time that you are unable to tolerate the pain, and the position changes recommended in the following pages do not help, consult a lactation professional. If none is available, you may want to stop nursing; pump your milk with a fully automatic electric pump for 24 to 72 hours, or until the nipples heal (see page 175 for information on expressing milk).

There are two basic types of sore nipples: the traumatized nipple and the irritated nipple. The traumatized nipple may be blistered, scabbed, or cracked. The irritated nipple is very pink and often burns. Occasionally a mother may have both types of soreness at once.

In addition to the specific treatments listed for each category of sore nipples, the "General Comfort Measures for Sore Nipples," below, will speed healing and provide comfort.

General Comfort Measures for Sore Nipples

1. Take acetaminophen tablets (such as Tylenol), ibuprofen (such as Advil or Motrin), or a pain reliever prescribed by your doctor, a half hour before nursing.
2. Begin nursing on the least sore side (if there is one).
3. Avoid nipple shields for nursing. These often make the soreness worse, and they may decrease your milk supply. If nursing is too painful, rent a fully automatic electric pump.
4. Massage your breasts while nursing to encourage the milk to flow and to speed emptying.
5. Restrict nursing time to about ten to fifteen minutes per side if you are sore during the entire feeding. This will probably mean nursing more often (every hour or two).
6. Release the baby's suction hold carefully before removing the baby from the breast.
7. Air-dry the nipples after each feeding. Leave the nipples exposed to the air as much as possible between nursings. A cotton T-shirt worn without a bra, or with your bra flaps down, will provide good air circulation to the nipples.
8. Change nursing pads after each nursing and when they become wet. Make sure there are no plastic liners hidden in the pads; cut them open and check if you are not absolutely sure.
9. Wear cotton or microfiber bras. Other fabrics do not allow adequate air circulation.
10. Wash plastic breast shells daily, if you use them at all. Shells may prevent the nipples from rubbing against your bra, but unless they are vented they may also encourage dripping, keep the nipples moist, and delay healing.
11. Avoid excessive washing of your nipples. Rinse them in your daily bath or shower, but avoid getting soap on them. Do take care to wash your hands before handling your breasts.
12. Leave scabs and blisters alone.
13. Do not delay nursings. Shorter, more frequent nursings (every hour to three hours) are easier on the nipples.

14. If you are using a breast pump during a period of soreness, pump your milk often—at least eight times a day—to keep up your supply. Again, anything other than a fully automatic pump (a rental pump) may not be effective enough to maintain your milk supply. Be sure to use the correct size shield for your nipple, and carefully center it before starting to pump (see page 175 for more information on expressing milk).

Traumatized nipples. Cracks, blisters, and abrasions usually result because a baby is improperly positioned for nursing; her gums close on the nipple instead of the areola. Trauma can also occur when a baby fails to open her mouth wide enough or when her gums slide off the areola onto the nipple, commonly when the breast is engorged or not supported.

Babies who have a faulty suck or who are "tongue-tied" can also make nipples sore as they nurse (see the section on "tongue-tied" babies on page 70). Cracking may also occur with irritated nipples and thrush nipples (see the sections on both).

Treatment Measures for Traumatized Nipples

1. Carefully review "Positioning at the Breast," pages 30–35, so that you clearly understand the details of correct latch-on technique. The football or the cross-over hold is highly recommended.

2. If your breast is so full that the areola cannot be easily compressed, manually express or pump enough milk to soften the areola. This will allow the baby to get more of the areola into her mouth and will help to stimulate let-down.

3. Use the football or the cross-over hold to control the position of the baby's head through the entire feeding. This will allow you to prevent her gums from sliding down onto the nipple after she has latched on.

4. If your baby is reluctant to open her mouth wide, don't let her chew her way onto the breast. Patiently wait until she opens her mouth wide. Letting the baby suck on your finger for a few seconds may stimulate her sucking response and encourage her to open more enthusiastically.

5. Do not hesitate to take the baby off the breast as soon as you realize that she is not in the right position. You may need to help her latch on several times before you succeed at getting her far enough onto the breast. Ask your partner, helper, or lactation professional to observe your latch-on

technique. A helper can also guide your arm when ~~opens~~ opens wide so that she is pulled in as close as pos~~sible~~

6. After nursing, apply a thin coating of modified lanolin ~~to~~ your nipples to soothe them and promote healing. You might also wear vented, hard plastic breast shells between nursings, to keep your bra off your sensitive nipples. Review "General Comfort Measures for Sore Nipples," page 51.

7. Try wearing hydrogel dressings between nursings. These cool, soothing pads, made of fluid-absorbing gel granules, may speed healing by keeping injured nipples moist enough to prevent scab formation but not excessively damp. Similar pads made with glycerin promote healing in the same fashion. See Appendix A, page 244, for information on locating these pads.

8. If you have a wound on your nipple that hasn't closed in five days, ask your midwife or doctor for oral antibiotics. The wound may be infected, and such an infection not only slows healing of the nipple but also puts a woman at high risk for developing mastitis in the coming weeks. Take the antibiotic for 10 to 14 days, or longer if healing isn't complete.

Irritated nipples. Irritated nipples are reddened and sometimes slightly swollen, and *generally they burn*. Some mothers may feel burning between as well as during feedings. In severe cases, the nipples may be cracked, peeling, or oozing. Irritated nipples may be caused by thrush or yeast, dermatitis, or an underlying skin condition such as eczema or impetigo.

Thrush nipples. This problem occurs when a yeast *(monilia)* infection in the baby's mouth spreads to the mother's nipples. The nipples become shiny, reddened, swollen, tender, and sometimes cracked. Occasionally peeling or a red, dotty rash can be seen on the nipples. Some mothers complain of itching and flaking; others complain of burning.

When a mother's nipples become sore after weeks or months of comfortable nursing, thrush is the usual cause. But a thrush infection may also occur in the first weeks after delivery, and when it does it may be overlooked as the cause of the nipple soreness. A newborn with thrush may have picked up a yeast infection in the birth canal during delivery; this often happens if the mother is diabetic. A thrush infection may also result if a mother or her baby is given antibiotics (after a cesarean, antibiotics are often given in intravenous fluids).

▶ *Thrush often appears as white, cheesy patches on the insides of the cheeks and lips.*

If you suspect a case of thrush, carefully inspect the baby's mouth. You may see white patches on the inside of the cheeks, inside the lips, and possibly on the tongue. Sometimes a baby will have no symptoms in the mouth but will have a diaper rash caused by yeast. This rash, usually in the genital area, often resembles a mild burn; it may peel and does not respond to ordinary measures. Sometimes the rash looks like just a patch of red dots.

Treatment Measures for Thrush Nipples

1. Both the mother and the baby must be treated in order to prevent reinfection. The treatment usually recommended is 1 milliliter of nystatin suspension (Mycostatin) by dropper into the baby's mouth after every other nursing, or four times daily, for 14 days. Half the dose should be dropped into each side of the mouth. For the nipples, nystatin cream or ointment is recommended; the baby's medicine can also be used, but it is often less effective. The medication should be applied after each nursing. In either form, nystatin must be prescribed by a physician. Even though the symptoms may be gone after a few days, continue the treatment for the full 14 days.

   Another medication that is sometimes recommended is a 1-percent solution of gentian violet, which can be purchased at most drugstores without a prescription. Thoroughly swab the affected areas in the baby's mouth with a cotton-tipped applicator once or twice a day for three days. The solution will stain the baby's mouth purple; take care in applying so that nothing else turns purple. Some lactation professionals recommend painting the mother's nipples with gentian violet, too, but I don't recommend this treatment for tender nipples.

If you cannot get your baby's doctor to prescribe nystatin cream for your nipples (and your baby's diaper rash, if present), call your obstetrician for a prescription, or use an over-the-counter antifungal cream such as Lotrimin AF, Micatin, or Monistat 7.

2. If you are using nystatin, it is best to wait for a few minutes after nursing before giving it to the baby so that it isn't washed out of his system with the milk. Some lactation professionals also recommend rinsing your nipples after each nursing the first few days with water or a mild solution of vinegar (one tablespoon vinegar to one cup water) before applying the cream or drops.

3. In addition to medication, brief exposure to the sun two or three times daily may hasten the healing of the nipples.

4. Changing the nursing pads at each feeding is a must to prevent reinfection.

5. Pacifiers, bottle nipples, and plastic breast shells must be boiled for 5 minutes every day during treatment. If you are using nystatin, these nipples should be replaced at the end of the first week.

6. If you are using a pump, it is important to wash all pump parts thoroughly after each use. In addition, the parts that come in contact with the breast or the milk should be boiled for 5 minutes daily.

7. If nystatin suspension has not cleared thrush from your baby's mouth after five to six days of treatment, consider that this medication inhibits yeast growth for only about two hours after you swab the baby's mouth. Ask your doctor about more frequent dosing, or try using gentian violet (as described in item 1) in addition to the nystatin.

8. Also consider trying fluconazole (Diflucan), an oral antifungal agent. The dosage usually prescribed is 200 milligrams on the first day followed by 100 milligrams for the next 13 days. This medication is terribly expensive, though, and I find most mothers can overcome yeast infections by using antifungal cream on the nipples and frequently treating the baby's mouth.

9. If your nipples aren't significantly better after several days of the treatment just described, see a dermatologist for additional treatment. In the absence of visible thrush, pink, burning nipples may indicate nipple dermatitis, a bacterial infection of the nipples, or both.

Nipple dermatitis. A slight reddening and a burning feeling in the nipples, in the absence of thrush (yeast) or another underlying skin condition, usually indicates dermatitis. Nipple dermatitis can result from bacterial growth on the nipples or an allergic response to a nipple cream, oil, or to laundry detergents.

Common offenders are vitamin E preparations—oils, creams, or capsules. Mothers allergic to chocolate may develop an allergic reaction to preparations with cocoa butter, such as Balm Barr. Unmodified lanolin may also cause an allergic response, usually in a mother who is allergic to wool (from which lanolin comes) or very sensitive to it. Lanolin is found in pure hydrous and anhydrous forms and in many commercial creams, such as Masse Cream, Mammol Ointment, Eucerin, and A & D Ointment. Modified lanolin, which has had the allergenic component removed, seldom causes allergic reactions.

Simply discontinuing use of the cream or oil, or switching to hypo-allergenic detergents (free of perfumes and dyes) may bring some relief, but usually additional measures are necessary.

Treatment Measures for Nipple Dermatitis

1. The ideal doctor to diagnose and treat this type of nipple soreness is a dermatologist. Usually, a moderate-strength or high-potency anti-inflammatory cream and an antibiotic cream are prescribed. Your obstetrician may give you a prescription, but if he is reluctant or his remedy is ineffective, see a dermatologist.
2. Place cool, wet compresses on the nipples after nursing.
3. Apply the medication to the irritated areas after every other nursing, making sure your nipples are completely dry first. The cream should be applied sparingly so that all of it is absorbed. If you see traces on your nipples when you are ready to nurse again, you are using too much. Dab the area with a tissue to absorb the excess.
4. Use the medication for as long as advised by your doctor. Although the pain may be gone in a day or two, the dermatitis may take from one to two weeks to completely heal.
5. Should you find that the medication aggravates your soreness, stop using it immediately. This may indicate that yeast is present and should be treated. (See "Thrush Nipples," page 53.)
6. Review "General Comfort Measures for Sore Nipples," page 51.

Eczema and impetigo. Eczema can appear on the nipple and areo making the area burn, itch, flake, ooze, or crust. Women with a his tory or current outbreak of eczema elsewhere on the body are most often affected. Treatment from a dermatologist should be sought.

Impetigo is a severe infection that causes continual sloughing off of the skin. Impetigo on the nipples can be quickly cured with a prescription antibiotic cream.

Breast pain

You may feel pain in your breasts if you become engorged, which usually happens two to four days after delivery (see "Engorged Breasts," page 48). Occasionally mothers complain of breast pain while nursing. If you feel a burning pain and your nipples are pinker than normal, see "Irritated Nipples," page 53. If you feel a mild aching at the start of nursing, it is probably related to the beginning of let-down.

A deep pain, sometimes described as "shooting," that occurs soon after nursing is believed to be related to the sudden refilling of the breast. This discomfort is usually temporary and disappears after the first weeks of nursing.

Leaking milk

During the early weeks of nursing, milk may drip, leak, or spray from the breasts. This is a normal sign of let-down. While the baby nurses at one breast, milk often drips or sprays from the other. Let-down, and leaking, may occur frequently and unexpectedly between nursings as well. Milk may leak during sleep. It may be stimulated by the baby's sounds, by thoughts about nursing, or by any routines associated with feeding time. A shower may stimulate let-down. Dripping, leaking, and spraying usually lessen considerably after a few weeks of nursing.

Some mothers' breasts do not leak. Women who have nursed previously may notice that their breasts leak less with subsequent children. Both of these situations are usually normal.

Coping Measures for Leaking Milk

1. Open both bra flaps while nursing and let the milk drip into a small towel or diaper.
2. Change cloth or disposable nursing pads as soon as they become wet. Avoid those with plastic liners.
3. Try silicone nursing pads, which don't absorb milk but instead apply a gentle pressure on the nipple to prevent

(See Appendix A, page 244, for information on how
silicone nursing pads.)

tine use of plastic breast shells if you do not need
prove the shape of your nipples. They may keep
...es dry, but they can cause excessive leaking and
keep your nipples moist. Milk collected in the shells between
nursings is unsafe for feeding. Only if the shells are boiled
just prior to nursing and put in place during nursing can the
milk be stored for later feedings.

5. Don't try to control leaking by habitually pumping your
breasts. Pumping actually stimulates greater milk production
and could make your breasts fuller and more prone to
leaking.

6. If your breasts leak during the night, place extra cloth or
disposable pads in your bra or use LilyPadz, which adhere
to the skin and don't require a bra to hold them in place.
(See Appendix A, page 244, for ordering information.) Or
spread a bath towel over the bed sheet to keep it and your
mattress dry.

Let-down difficulty

During the early weeks of breastfeeding, the
let-down response is developing. Sometimes
mothers are told that they must be happy,
relaxed, and carefree for the let-down of milk to occur. If this were
the case, few women would ever succeed at nursing. Although many
mothers worry that their milk won't be available as needed, let-down
failure is extremely rare among women who nurse regularly and
often.

For the establishment and maximal functioning of the let-down
reflex, nurse the baby every two to three hours around the clock
during the first week. Make sure that she is positioned correctly and
is compressing the sinuses beneath the areola, and that her feeding
time is not limited. Ideally, the baby should be allowed—encouraged,
if necessary—to drain one or both breasts well at each feeding.

It is also important that you are as comfortable as possible. The
milk may not release completely if you are experiencing much pain—
whether from sore nipples or from the trauma of delivery.

The signs of milk release during the first week will vary for each
woman. They *may* include—

● mild uterine cramping during nursing;

● increased vaginal flow during nursing;

- dripping, leaking, or spraying of milk, especially during nursing;

- occasional sensations in the breast during nursing (usually not felt during the first week); and

- softening of the breasts after nursing.

The most reliable indicator of milk let-down is the sound of the baby swallowing. As the milk releases, the baby will swallow after every one or two sucks. Most women, particularly first-time mothers, do not feel the let-down reflex during the first few weeks after birth.

Usually when a mother believes she is experiencing a let-down difficulty, the problem is actually with the baby's latch-on or sucking, or a low milk supply. See "Difficult Latch-on: Refusal to Nurse," page 68; "Sucking Problems," page 73; and "Underfeeding and Weight Loss," page 76, for more information on adequate milk supply.

Milk appearance

Whereas colostrum is usually clear, yellow, or orange, mature breast milk is white, sometimes with a bluish tint. If it resembles skim milk from the dairy, this does not mean your milk is "weak"; breast milk normally looks thin. Occasionally a mother discovers that her milk is green, blue, or pink. Such coloring is due to her intake of vegetables, fruits, food dyes, or dietary supplements, and is not harmful to the baby.

Blood in the milk can usually be traced to a bleeding nipple. Occasionally, bleeding from the breast occurs during pregnancy or when breastfeeding begins. Frequently, a benign papilloma is the cause, and the bleeding generally stops within several days. Blood in the milk will not hurt the baby, though substantial amounts may make him vomit. If you are advised against nursing, pump for a few days. The problem will clear up on its own in a day or so.

Difficult latch-on: Flat, dimpled, or inverted nipples

Both mother and baby get frustrated when latching on to the breasts is difficult because of flat, dimpled, or inverted nipples. Typically, the problem is intensified if the breasts become engorged or overly full. When they do, even nipples that seemed normal may suddenly flatten or dimple. Frequently, one nipple proves to be more troublesome than the other. Persistence and patience help most mothers through this problem.

Mothers with problem nipples are often more prone to soreness. This is because latch-on becomes their number-one priority; they give little attention to correct positioning.

Treatment Measures for Flat, Dimpled, or Inverted Nipples

1. Put the baby to the breast within the first two hours after birth. The timing of the first nursing may be critical when the nipples are flat, dimpled, or inverted. Many babies are able to latch on easily to problem nipples during this initial period, and they continue to do well.

2. Avoid giving the baby an artificial nipple of any kind. Whether or not your baby has succeeded at latching on at first try, this is very important. An artificial nipple often makes his subsequent attempts more difficult.

3. Stimulate the nipples to help them stand out, by gently stroking or rolling them between your thumb and forefinger or by applying ice to the nipple just before the baby attempts to latch on.

4. To help the baby latch on to a flat nipple, make it stand out by pinching it between your thumb and forefinger. This won't work with a dimpled or inverted nipple, though; it may invert further when pinched. To help the baby latch on to an inverted or dimpled nipple, place your thumb about 1½ to 2 inches behind the nipple, with your fingers beneath, and pull back toward your chest. The cross-over or football hold will allow you the most visibility and control.

5. Wear breast shells in your bra at least a half-hour before nursing if your breasts are engorged; this is often essential for dimpled or inverted nipples. Many hospital maternity units have breast shells. If yours doesn't, send your partner or friend to any maternity shop for a pair. (See "Planning for the First Days," page 15.)

6. Pump your breasts just before nursing to pull the nipples out enough for the baby to latch on. Any pump can be used for this.

▲ *To help the baby latch on to an inverted nipple, place your thumb above the areola and your fingers below, and push your breast against your chest wall.*

▲ *Don't squeeze your thumb and forefinger together, or the nipple may invert further.*

7. Express a few drops of colostrum or milk onto your nipple or onto the baby's lips if he is reluctant to latch on. Glucose water (available only in hospital nurseries) dripped over the nipple may also entice the baby, although it sometimes makes the nipple too slippery. At home, in a pinch, you can mix a teaspoon of refined sugar in a cup of warm boiled water, then drip the solution over your nipple. But *never* use honey or corn syrup on your nipple, as they have been associated with infant botulism.

8. Stop nursing if the baby is frantic, and calm him for a while. Dripping glucose water on his lips also helps to calm him and gain his interest in latching on.

9. If a nurse or another helper is working with you, use the side-lying position—or, if you're large-breasted, the football hold—to allow your helper maximum visibility and control. If your nipples are dimpled or inverted, ask the helper to pull back on the breast behind the nipple; pinching will usually result in further inversion. Sometimes these sessions become intense and upsetting, so let your helper know when you or your baby needs a break. If you are in the hospital, let a variety of nurses work with you; you can usually find one or two who are exceptionally skilled and sensitive.

10. Refuse any offers from nurses of rubber nipple shields or bottle nipples to place over your own nipple for nursing. Your baby will latch on and suck, but the shield may not allow for adequate stimulation of your nipple, or for the necessary compression of the sinuses beneath the areola. The shield can thus inhibit the let-down of milk and adequate emptying of the breast, possibly leading to a poor milk supply and insufficient milk intake for the baby. In addition, some babies who begin nursing with a nipple shield will refuse to ever nurse without it.

   If you want to try using a nipple shield to make your nipples stand out, wait at least 24 hours after the birth, to give the baby a chance to nurse on his own. Take the shield off after the baby has sucked for one to two minutes, and try to get him to latch on without it. Pumping just before nursing may work just as well as a nipple shield in making the nipples stand out.

   Use a nipple shield throughout feedings only if (1) a lactation professional makes sure that the baby is taking enough milk while you're wearing the shield, or (2) you use a fully automatic electric pump after each nursing to guarantee that your breasts are being well emptied, and you have the baby weighed every few days to make sure he is gaining at least an ounce a day.

11. Begin bottle feedings 24 hours after birth if your baby still has not latched on. An electric pump is usually the best choice for collecting milk and improving the nipple shape. Continue putting the baby to breast.

12. Occasionally a mother and her baby are discharged from the hospital before nursing has occurred. If this happens to you, locate a fully automatic electric pump (see Appendix A, page 243) and use it at least eight times a day. (See page 98 for guidelines on pumping exclusively, and refer to Appendix B, page 252, for the approximate amount of milk your baby needs at each feeding.) Keep trying to nurse; once at home, short practice sessions at least three to four times per day, on a soft breast when the baby is not frantic, eventually pay off. In this situation you may need a great deal of support and encouragement. Finding this support will make all the difference. Seeing a lactation professional may be very helpful. It is very common for a baby to suddenly latch on one day, rewarding his mother's persistence.

Fatigue and depression

During this first week, make your life as simple as possible. Your partner or helper is essential, of course, to your recovery and adjustment. He or she can be most helpful in assuring your rest by taking over family and household duties and limiting phone calls and visitors.

Rest is necessary to your ability to cope during the postpartum period. Make a commitment to take at least one nap a day, to make up for sleep lost in labor and afterward, due to frequent feeding demands. You may find that you are able to sleep better during naps and at night if you tuck the baby in with you. Babies often sleep better this way, too. An answering machine can be very helpful in preventing disruptions while you nap. It's also handy when you are busy with nursing and baby care.

Eat a good breakfast—perhaps your partner can prepare it for you. If you lack an appetite at mealtimes, frequent snacking throughout the day on high-protein foods will assist your own physical recovery and help maintain your energy level.

If you have had tearing or an episiotomy, or you have hemorrhoids, take several baths each day. Warm water is soothing and relaxing, and it will speed the healing of your perineum.

Don't expect yourself to adjust to new parenthood on your own. Reach out for help or reassurance whenever you need it. Friends or relatives might welcome the opportunity to come and help out for a while, and you should feel free to call the hospital staff, a public health nurse, your childbirth instructor, or a breastfeeding counselor whenever you need assistance, reassurance, or support.

If you feel tired and overwhelmed, try not to keep it to yourself. Let your partner know—a good cry on someone's shoulder may leave you feeling much better. Avoid making your partner the target of your fears and anger; instead of criticizing, let him know exactly what you need. One mother put it very well: "I just need him to give me hugs and let me know I'm doing OK." Your partner, after all, may be feeling as much stress as you are.

Feeling depressed over a birth experience is not uncommon. You may be able to resolve some of your feelings by talking to your childbirth instructor or birth attendant. In a week or two, you might try to locate a postpartum or cesarean support group.

If you are alone with your baby during this first week, make a special effort to continue limiting your activities. Perhaps you can have a friend come by to fix you lunch. Let the dishes soak all day, and pick up the house for only ten minutes at a time, if you must. Unplug the phone and place a sign on your door when it's time for your nap. Perhaps you can afford to pay for light housekeeping once or twice a week for a short period.

CONCERNS ABOUT THE BABY

Sleepy baby

Most babies are sleepy during the first several days after birth. They may be so sleepy that they refuse to nurse or they fall asleep after just a few minutes of nursing. Sleepiness during the first few days may be related in part to recovery following labor and delivery. Pain medications and general anesthetics given to the mother during the birth process also lessen the baby's wakefulness and interest in nursing. When newborns are wrapped snugly, too, they usually sleep for long periods of time (that's why nurses bundle them tightly). Babies may act too sleepy to nurse when they feel full from water or formula supplements—or an air bubble. The newborn with jaundice may also be somewhat sleepy.

Although it may seem unkind, the sleepy baby should be wakened and fed at least every three hours. The sleepy baby needs a "mother-led" rather than a "demand" schedule until she begins waking on her own. This is necessary not only for her nutritional well-being but to ensure milk production and supply. Frequent feedings will also help minimize jaundice.

Treatment Measures for the Sleepy Baby

1. Attempt nursing only after waking the baby. This is best accomplished by unwrapping and undressing her down to the diaper. Dim any bright lights, and sit the baby up on your lap by holding her under her chin. While talking to the baby, gently rub or pat her back (you may even get a burp).
2. Stroke the baby's forehead with a cool (not cold) washcloth to help waken the very persistent sleeper.
3. If the baby falls back asleep soon after latching on, use the side-lying position to encourage her to nurse for longer periods. You may need assistance from someone else to get the baby to latch on. The football hold may also be helpful in keeping the baby awake, though not as effective as side-lying nursing.
4. Burp the baby after nursing at one breast to encourage her to take the other. Sitting the baby up in your lap and bending her slightly forward usually works best. Change her diaper if needed.
5. Be persistent. If all else fails, which may happen, try again in a half hour.
6. Avoid supplements, pacifiers, and nipple shields. All of these may increase the baby's reluctance to nurse.
7. While in the hospital, take advantage of the baby's normal sleeping and waking cycles by keeping her with you as much as possible.
8. Alert your physician if your baby is very lethargic and cannot be roused by the preceding techniques after five to six hours.

Bowel movements

Your baby's first few stools are called meconium. Meconium is black, greenish-black, or dark brown, and is tarry or sticky. By the second or third day, after several good colostrum feedings, the baby will have passed most of the meconium; he may have a few greenish-brown or brownish-yellow transitional stools.

Once milk production is established and the baby is nursing well, stools take on their characteristic yellow or mustard color. This usually occurs by the fifth day, unless the baby is jaundiced and is receiving phototherapy, which makes the stools dark, or he is not getting enough milk. Yellow stools by the fifth day are a sign that the baby is getting sufficient milk.

During the early days most babies have at least a few bowel movements daily. The stools of a breastfed baby are generally the consistency of yogurt. They are soft and may even be runny; they may appear curdled or seedy. This is not diarrhea. These stools have a sweet or cheesy odor.

Your baby may pass his stools easily, or he may fuss, grunt, and turn red in the face while having a bowel movement. This is not constipation. Constipation is not possible as long as your baby is totally breastfed.

If your baby doesn't have bowel movements every day, or if by the fifth day his stools are still dark, he may not be getting enough milk. See "Underfeeding and Weight Loss," page 76, for more information on how to determine if your baby is getting enough.

Jaundice

A yellowing of the skin and eyes, jaundice is caused by bilirubin, a yellow pigment that is present to some degree in all blood. The skin becomes yellowish when the amount of bilirubin is higher than normal.

Bilirubin comes from the red blood cells. These cells live only a short time; as they are destroyed, bilirubin is made. Bilirubin is then processed through the liver and finally eliminated in the stool. During pregnancy, the mother's liver processes bilirubin for the baby. After birth, the baby's liver has to learn to do the job. This usually takes a few days. Until the baby's liver is able to process bilirubin, it may increase in the baby's blood. This normal rise is referred to as physiologic jaundice. This is the most common form of jaundice, and about 40 percent of all babies develop it. It is usually noticed on the second or third day of life, and it generally disappears by one week of age.

Mild to moderate jaundice of this type will not hurt a baby, although many parents worry about it. However, the baby who nurses poorly or not at all during the first few days may become jaundiced from the lack of colostrum, which is important for the elimination of meconium. When meconium is retained in the bowel longer than usual, bilirubin cannot be eliminated as needed. The best way to treat this jaundice is to make sure the baby gets plenty of colostrum and breast milk (see "Underfeeding and Weight Loss," page 76).

Some babies develop jaundice for other reasons. One type of jaundice, ABO incompatibility, occurs when the mother's blood type is O and the baby's blood type is A, B, or AB. During pregnancy, maternal antibodies cross the placenta, break down red blood cells, and cause more bilirubin to be produced in the baby after birth. On the first or second day after delivery, the bilirubin level may rise rapidly. Other, less common blood incompatibilities also produce elevated bilirubin levels. Babies of East Asian descent typically experience higher bilirubin levels.

Babies with any bruises resulting from the birth process commonly develop jaundice. Also more prone to jaundice are babies who are sick right after birth or born prematurely, at low birth weights, or to diabetic mothers. Twins, too, are especially susceptible. Some drugs that are used during labor, including pitocin, can also cause jaundice.

Another type of jaundice, known as breast-milk jaundice, occurs in approximately one-third of all nursing babies. Breast-milk jaundice does not generally appear until the fifth day after birth. It usually

▲ *Nurse often during phototherapy; taking the baby from under the bili-light for feedings will not slow her recovery from jaundice.*

lasts four to six weeks but can continue for as long as eight to ten weeks. The exact cause of this jaundice is still unknown, but it has never been known to cause any problem for a baby. When a baby's skin stays yellow beyond the first week, breast-milk jaundice is diagnosed by laboratory tests that rule out other forms of jaundice. Breastfeeding need not be interrupted to make this diagnosis.

If your baby looks jaundiced, the doctor may order tests to measure the level of bilirubin in the blood and determine whether treatment is necessary. If the baby was born at term and is otherwise healthy, many doctors will not order treatment unless the bilirubin level is over 20 milligrams per deciliter. Frequent breastfeeding may be all that is necessary.

Some babies may be treated with phototherapy. The "bili-lights," along with frequent nursing, help to destroy excess bilirubin. The baby usually lies under these lights from two to four days, her eyes covered with a protective mask. Often, the bilirubin level will stay constant for 24 hours and drop by 48 hours. The treatment is discontinued as soon as the bilirubin level has dropped to a normal level. Usually a baby is hospitalized for phototherapy, but in some communities home phototherapy services are available.

Rarely, usually in cases of blood incompatibility, the bilirubin climbs rapidly to high levels. On these occasions an exchange transfusion may be done to reduce the bilirubin. Over an hour or two, small amounts of the baby's blood are taken out and replaced with donated blood.

Some doctors ask the mother to stop breastfeeding temporarily whenever a baby becomes jaundiced. This is generally unwise, since breastfeeding is usually one of the most effective ways of eliminating jaundice. Calling a halt to nursing is also unfortunate for the mother, who may wonder if her milk is really best for her baby.

Mothers are also commonly told that their nursing babies need water supplements to help get rid of jaundice. Water supplements do not lower the level of bilirubin in the blood. Some studies suggest that water supplements are associated with higher bilirubin levels. Moreover, babies who are routinely given water tend to be nursed less frequently, and they have a higher rate of early weaning.

Since 1994, the American Academy of Pediatrics has recommended a different approach: Healthy, full-term babies over 72 hours old with bilirubin levels below 20 milligrams per deciliter (or 340 micromoles per liter) should be nursed frequently, at least eight times every 24 hours, and should receive no water supplements.

Treatment Measures for Jaundice

1. Let the baby's physician know you prefer to continue nursing throughout the period of jaundice.

2. Nurse frequently, ideally every two to two and a half hours, and encourage the baby to suck at least 15 to 20 minutes at each breast. If your baby needs phototherapy, taking her from under the bili-light for these feedings will not delay the effectiveness of treatment. Intermittent phototherapy is thought to be as effective as continuous exposure.

3. If your baby is sleepy, as jaundiced babies sometimes are, see "Sleepy Baby," page 63, for effective measures on how to wake her up.

4. Avoid water supplements, as these do not reduce bilirubin levels and may discourage the baby from nursing frequently.

5. To be sure your baby is getting enough milk, keep track of her bowel movements. She should have at least a few each day. She should have lost less than 10 percent of her birth weight, and she should gain an ounce a day after the fifth day. If she doesn't gain this much, refer to "Underfeeding and Weight Loss," page 76.

6. If you are still hospitalized or you are welcome to stay in a hospital room while your baby is being treated, ask the nurses if you can have the baby's crib and light set up next to your bed so you can care for the baby and nurse frequently.

7. If you cannot stay 24 hours a day with your baby, express your milk every three hours (see page 175). Take your milk to the hospital for the feedings you will miss.

8. If your doctor is firm in her desire for you to temporarily stop nursing, again, express milk every three hours to keep your supply up. Freeze your milk and save it for later. In this case a fully automatic electric pump is strongly recommended (see Appendix A, page 243).

Difficult latch-on: Refusal to nurse

Latch-on problems can originate with the baby or the mother. Most occur when the baby is sleepy (see "Sleepy Baby," page 63); when the breast becomes overly full or engorged (see "Engorged Breasts," page 48); when the mother and baby are not positioned well for latch-on; or when the mother has flat, dimpled, or inverted nipples (see "Difficult Latch-on: Flat, Dimpled, or Inverted Nipples," page 59). Problems other than these are as follows.

The baby who has nursed earlier. During the first week, it is not uncommon for a baby who has already nursed to suddenly refuse one or both sides. He may simply act uninterested although he is awake, or he may protest furiously when put to one or both breasts. A baby who has been given a bottle or pacifier during the first week may become "nipple-confused" and refuse to nurse thereafter. Such a baby will likely start nursing again after a few hours uncoaxed or after one or more of the following measures are taken.

Treatment Measures for the Baby Who Stops Nursing

1. Soften the areola if you are overly full or engorged by using manual expression or a pump just before putting the baby to breast.
2. Calm the frantic baby. A few drops of colostrum or glucose water (available only in hospital nurseries) on his lips or dripped over the nipple will often alert and encourage him. At home, in a pinch, you can mix a teaspoon of refined sugar in a cup of warm boiled water to entice the baby. Occasionally a very upset baby may need to be tightly swaddled in a thin blanket.
3. Pay attention to proper positioning (see "Positioning at the Breast," page 30). When the baby turns his face from side to side with mouth wide open, pull him in closer so his tongue can feel the nipple.
4. Try letting the baby suck on your finger for a few seconds just before putting him to breast.
5. If the baby seems to spit out the nipple with his tongue, try holding some ice against the nipple for a few minutes to firm it. This can be particularly effective for the baby who acts "nipple-confused."
6. Persist. The baby who is hiccoughing, having a bowel movement, or staring at his mother or something else interesting will usually be reluctant to latch on. Try again in a half hour or so.
7. Coax the baby who is suddenly refusing one breast by using the football hold on that side.
8. If you can't get the baby latched on, express your milk until you can. Refer to Appendix B, page 252, for the approximate amounts of milk a baby needs at each feeding.

The baby who has not yet nursed. If a day or more has passed since the baby's birth and she still has not managed to latch on and suck, she probably has one of the specific problems described as follows.

Recessed jaw. Some babies are born with a very recessed lower jaw. This can best be seen by looking at the baby's face in profile. A recessed jaw is problematic because a baby can latch on only if her chin reaches the breast before her upper lip; otherwise she can't take enough breast tissue into her mouth.

When you try to get a baby like this to latch on, make sure your breast isn't overly full. Extend the baby's head slightly backward as you bring her onto the breast, so that her chin touches the breast first. Most babies overcome this problem by four to six weeks of age, when they are finally able to latch on and suck efficiently. In the meantime, you may need to pump your milk and feed it to your baby by bottle.

Tongue-tied. Some of the infants in this situation—mostly males— are tongue-tied. The frenulum, or string-like tissue that attaches to the underside of the tongue, is so short or connected so close to the tip of the tongue that the baby may not be able to extend his tongue past his bottom lip. Although he can suck on a finger or rubber nipple that extends well into his mouth, he may be unable to grasp the underside of his mother's nipple. Occasionally, a tongue-tied baby can manage to latch on to one breast but not the other.

The solution is simple: the frenulum should be clipped to release the tongue. However, some physicians are reluctant or unwilling to perform this procedure, because studies conducted several years ago showed that tongue-tied

▲ *The tongue-tied baby may not be able to extend his tongue far enough to latch on to his mother's nipple.*

infants rarely develop speech difficulties later in life; the studies concluded that tongue clipping was therefore unnecessary. Unfortunately, though, some tongue-tied babies are unable to breastfeed. If you cannot persuade your doctor to clip the frenulum, find another who will. An experienced surgeon or dentist may do this in his or her office. The procedure takes just a minute.

Tongue thrusting (nipple confusion). Some babies push their tongues forward while trying to latch on or suck, and by doing so they spit the nipple out. Babies may do this from birth or as a result of sucking on a rubber nipple. When a rubber nipple is to blame, the problem is referred to as nipple confusion. Tongue-thrusting babies can usually relearn to nurse, with some assistance.

Protruding tongue. A few babies have tongues that protrude. The tongue may look longer than normal; it may be visible between the lips much of the time. Some mothers have described the protruding tongue as forming a hump in the mouth that the nipple is not able to get past.

You may be able to teach the baby to nurse by encouraging her to open wide with her tongue down and pulling back behind the areola just before latch-on. The football hold is recommended for the best visibility and control. If you manage to get the baby on the breast, be sure she is sucking adequately. This means she does not come off the breast easily; is making long, drawing sucks; and is audibly swallowing. A few babies suck with the nipple in the front of the mouth; they rarely swallow and get very little milk.

Tongue sucking. Other infants who have difficulty latching on to the breast are those who suck their own tongues. These babies usually slide off the nipple after one or two sucks, and their cheeks dimple with each suck. They may also make clicking noises. When the baby opens her mouth to root or to cry, you may notice that her tongue is far back in her mouth or is curled toward the roof of her mouth.

Attempt to get the baby to latch on only when she opens wide with her tongue down. Stimulating the lower lip or slightly depressing the chin may help the tongue to drop. Pull the baby in very close.

▶ *Dimpling of the baby's cheeks during nursing may signify an inadequate suck.*

The cross-over or football hold is best when you are working alone, and side-lying will give more control and visibility when someone is assisting you.

When refusal persists. If you have followed the preceding suggestions and your baby still has not latched on, try the following measures.

Treatment Measures for Refusal to Nurse

1. Continue working with the baby. Short, frequent sessions may be less upsetting for both of you. If someone is working with you, the side-lying position may give her the greatest control and visibility. These sessions can become intense and sometimes upsetting, so let your helper know if you or the baby needs a break. If you are in the hospital, let several nurses work with you; you may find one or two who are exceptionally skilled and sensitive.

2. Refuse any offers from nurses of nipple shields or bottle nipples to place over your own nipple for nursing. Your baby will latch on and suck, but the shield may not allow for adequate nipple stimulation or for the necessary compression of the sinuses beneath the areola. This can seriously hamper the let-down of milk and adequate emptying of the breast, which may lead to a poor milk supply and insufficient intake for the baby. In addition, some babies will refuse ever to nurse without the shield. Use a nipple shield for entire feedings only if (1) a lactation professional is making sure that the baby is getting enough milk during feedings with the shield, or (2) you use a fully automatic electric pump after each nursing to guarantee that your breasts are being well emptied, and you have the baby weighed every few days to make sure he is gaining at least an ounce daily.

3. If after 24 hours your baby has not latched on, supplementary feedings should begin. Express your milk at least eight times a day, and feed the expressed milk to your baby.

4. If you are discharged from the hospital and your baby is still not nursing, use a fully automatic electric pump (see Appendix A, page 243) and keep giving pumped milk to the baby (see page 98 for guidelines on pumping). Refer to Appendix B, page 252, for the approximate amounts a baby needs at each feeding.

5. Continue short practice sessions several times a day. Some babies do better on a soft or empty breast.
6. Get lots of support and encouragement. If possible, see a lactation professional.
7. Be patient and persistent. Many babies with latch-on problems do overcome them sometime during the first ten days, but a significant number first latch on at about one month of age.

| Sucking problems |

Some babies can latch on to the breast but have a faulty sucking pattern. With some, the suction is so poor that they easily slide off the breast or can be taken off effortlessly. When they are nursing, their cheeks dimple with each suck, and frequent clicking noises may be audible. Most of these babies are sucking not on the nipple but on their tongues, which may perhaps be a habit developed in the uterus. These babies receive only the milk that drips into their mouths.

Although most babies with this problem have it from birth, others may develop it if they lose much weight, usually close to a pound, by the end of the first week. If this happens, and the baby cannot correct her suck after several good attempts at latching on, pump your milk and bottle-feed for 24 to 72 hours, supplementing breast milk with formula as necessary. After the baby is rehydrated and has regained a few ounces, she will probably correct her suck on her own.

A baby may have difficulty sucking at one or both breasts because she is tongue-tied. No matter how hard she tries, she may fail to get milk from the breast, and the mother's nipples may hurt even when the baby is correctly positioned. Sometimes a clicking sound can be heard as the baby sucks. To correct such a problem, have your doctor or dentist clip the baby's frenulum. (See the section on tongue-tied babies on page 70.)

Another group of babies who have difficulty sucking and getting enough milk are those with very high palates. When the roof of the mouth is very high, the baby has trouble compressing the breast against the palate to express the milk into her mouth. Many babies with high, arched palates do little swallowing at the breast and fail to gain weight well. Few health professionals, including pediatricians, yet recognize high palates as a potential problem for nursing babies. If it is difficult to see the very top of a baby's palate without placing your head close to the baby's chest, or if the shape of the roof looks much deeper than the curve of a teaspoon, the palate may be too high. If you can get the baby to suck on your little finger (nail side down), and you feel a frequent loss of suction between your finger and his tongue, or your finger isn't in firm contact with the roof of his mouth, the palate may be too high. Some babies with high palates are also tongue-tied.

In the case of a high palate, the only remedy I know of is for the mother to use an electric pump right after each nursing to bolster her milk supply. After a few days the baby will usually start to swallow more at the breast and gain weight better, but as soon as the pumping stops the baby begins to take less milk and will again fail to gain sufficient weight. Usually supplemental pumping is necessary for several weeks, until the baby has grown enough to suck more efficiently. Using the football hold may help the baby suck better.

Treatment Measures for the Baby with Poor Suction

1. Remove the baby from the breast as soon as this pattern is evident.
2. Observe the position of the tongue when the baby's mouth is wide open. If it is curled against the roof of the mouth, try to lower it with your finger. Sometimes touching the lower lip or pressing slightly on the chin will help.
3. Using the cross-over or football hold, pull the baby in as close as possible for latch-on.
4. Continue working with the baby. Short, frequent sessions may be less upsetting for both of you. If someone is working with you, the side-lying position may give her the greatest control and visibility. These sessions can become intense and upsetting, so let your helper know if you or the baby needs a break. If you are in the hospital, have several nurses work with you; you may find one or two who are exceptionally skilled and sensitive.
5. Refuse any offers from nurses of nipple shields or bottle nipples to place over your own nipple for nursing. Your baby will latch on and suck, but the shield may not allow for adequate nipple stimulation or for the necessary compression of the sinuses beneath the areola. This can seriously hamper the let-down of milk and adequate emptying of the breast, which may lead to a poor milk supply and insufficient intake for the baby. In addition, some babies will refuse ever to nurse without the shield. Use a nipple shield for entire feedings only if (1) a lactation professional makes sure that the baby is getting enough milk while you're wearing the shield, or (2) you use a fully automatic electric pump

after each nursing to guarantee that your breasts are being well emptied, and you have the baby weighed every few days to make sure he is gaining at least an ounce a day.

6. If after 24 hours your baby still has not latched on with strong suction, supplementary feedings should begin. Express your milk at least eight times a day, and feed the baby the expressed milk.

7. If you are discharged from the hospital and your baby still is not nursing, use a fully automatic electric pump (see Appendix A, page 243) and keep giving your milk to the baby (see page 98 for guidelines on pumping, and Appendix B, page 252, for the approximate amount of milk your baby needs at each feeding).

8. Continue short practice sessions several times a day. Some babies do better on a soft or empty breast.

9. Get lots of support and encouragement. If possible, see a lactation professional.

10. Be patient and persist. Many babies with sucking problems do overcome them sometime during the first ten days, but a significant number improve at about one month of age.

Fussiness and excessive night waking	It can come as a surprise when your baby suddenly becomes fussy after spending most of his first few days sleeping. It is difficult to listen to your baby's cry; it may feel like an alarm going

off in your body. Sometimes parents are told it is healthy for babies to cry, or that they will become spoiled if tended to every time they fuss. Comforting your infant and responding to her needs is very important to her well-being and her development of trust. Babies are really unspoilable.

Newborns cry for a variety of reasons. Often they are fussy their first night home from the hospital. They may be hungry as often as every hour, especially when the milk is just starting to come in, or when feedings have been limited because of their sleepiness or for other reasons. Some babies seem to need more sucking time than others. Some seem to pass a lot of gas, which causes them discomfort. Many newborns become upset when they are not kept snugly wrapped. Perhaps they miss the close, secure feeling of the womb.

Then there are the babies who sleep most of the day and wake frequently during the night. These babies are said to have their days and nights mixed up.

Coping Measures for Fussiness

1. Nurse your baby on demand, or at least every two to three hours for at least 15 to 20 minutes at each breast.
2. Massage your breasts while you nurse to encourage the milk to let down.
3. Burp the baby after he finishes at each breast. This will help prevent swallowed air from passing through the intestines and encourage him to nurse longer. If your baby is passing a lot of gas, you may need to burp him a few times during each feeding. See page 36 if you are having difficulty burping the baby.
4. Burp your baby after he uses a pacifier. Avoid using stuffed bottle nipples as pacifiers as these cause excessive air swallowing.
5. Wrap the baby snugly in a light blanket after feeding.
6. Avoid water or formula supplements. Perhaps you have nursed your baby but he acts as if he is still hungry. You can, certainly, offer him the breast again. But sometimes newborn babies will stay awake after a feeding and behave as if they need to suck longer even though their bellies are full. If the baby frequently seems unsatisfied, refer to "Underfeeding and Weight Loss," below. Most young infants will take water or formula if it is offered, even when they have had enough breast milk, but supplementing often leads to problems.

    If your baby does not seem content after nursing, feel free to nurse him some more, or try comforting him next to your body. Rocking or walking with the baby for a while will probably keep him content. In an hour or two, nurse him again.

Coping Measures for Excessive Night Waking

1. Nurse your baby every two to two and a half hours during the daytime and evening. If the baby is sleeping through feeding times, see "Sleepy Baby," page 63.
2. Tuck your baby in with you for at least a few nights; she may sleep better.

| **Underfeeding and weight loss** | During the first week, you may wonder if your baby is getting enough to eat. You may worry about whether the milk is adequate—espe- |

cially if the baby seems to be nursing all the time or is fussy after feedings. Some mothers wonder if their milk has dried up when they observe the normal softening of the breast that occurs as the initial engorgement recedes.

Seeing if the baby will take a bottle of water or formula after nursing is not a reliable method of determining if he is getting enough breast milk. Most babies will take a couple of ounces of water or formula if it is offered, even when they have had enough milk from the breast.

A baby can lose too much weight, though, when the milk doesn't come in by the third or fourth day, when nursing is infrequent, or when he has had trouble latching on and nursing well during the period of initial engorgement. Excessive weight loss can also occur when a mother uses a nipple shield over her nipple for nursing, when a newborn has a faulty suck, and, certainly, when a baby is sick. Sometimes laxatives the mother has taken can cause a baby to have excessive bowel movements and to lose weight or gain too slowly.

Signs of adequate milk intake are listed on page 38. If you and your baby don't show all these signs, have him weighed. If you find that your baby has lost 10 percent or more of his birth weight within the first five days after birth, or if he isn't gaining an ounce per day after the fifth day, take the following measures.

Treatment Measures for Underfeeding

1. If possible, see a lactation professional.
2. To estimate the amount of milk you are producing and to increase your milk supply, obtain a fully automatic electric breast pump (see Appendix A, page 243, for rental information). Any other pump would be inadequate for accurately estimating milk production and would be less helpful in increasing a low milk supply.
3. Estimate your milk production by pumping your breasts instead of nursing. If you are pumping one breast at a time, pump each breast twice, for a total pumping time of 20 to 25 minutes. If you have a double-pump collection kit, use it for a total of 12 to 15 minutes. Feed this milk and any necessary formula to your baby (see Appendix B, page 252, to determine how much milk your baby needs at each feeding). Exactly two hours after the completion of this pumping, pump again. You may very well get less milk at this second pumping than at the first. Multiply the number of ounces collected at the *second* pumping by 12. This will give you an estimate of how much milk you are producing over a 24-hour period; if you collect $1^{1}/_{2}$ ounces, for example, you are producing about 18 ounces per day.

4. If you determine that you have enough milk for your baby and yet she has not been gaining well, it may be that she is not taking all of the milk available at some or many of her feedings. This can happen with newborns who were born prematurely, who tend to drift off to sleep while nursing, or who have sucking difficulties.

5. After you have estimated your milk production, go back to nursing your baby. Be sure to nurse her at least eight times in every 24 hours. This may mean waking her for feedings. Wake a sleepy baby every two and a half hours (measured from the start of one nursing to the start of the next) during the day and evening, and every three to four hours in the night. Nurse your baby for 10 to 15 minutes at each breast. Frequent nursings of moderate duration are more effective in increasing milk production than lengthy but infrequent nursings.

6. Pump your breasts right after each nursing to stimulate further milk production. Unless you have a double-pump kit, pump each breast for five minutes, then return to each breast a second time for a few more minutes. Pumping both breasts at the same time is more effective in stimulating increased milk production and also takes less time. Use a double-pump kit for 5 to 10 minutes after nursing.

7. After pumping, feed the baby whatever breast milk you've collected along with any necessary formula. If the baby needs supplemental formula, divide the amount of supplement needed daily by the number of feedings the baby is getting each day (usually eight). A baby who needs $3\frac{1}{2}$ ounces of formula, for example, should get about $\frac{1}{2}$ ounce after each of her eight daily nursings. The goal is to offer about the same amount of breast milk and formula at each feeding so that the baby wants to nurse at regular intervals.

8. Consider using fenugreek to stimulate greater milk production. Fenugreek is a fragrant seed that is used as the flavoring ingredient in artificial maple syrup. You can make a tea from the seeds, but more convenient and effective is the capsule form, which is available in most health-food stores. Mothers who take two to three capsules three times a day typically notice an increase in the milk supply within one to three days. Although fenugreek capsules are usually used for just several days, some mothers have continued to use them for weeks or months without any difficulties. Fenugreek capsules cost about seven dollars for a bottle of 100.

Fenugreek is generally harmless, although you will probably notice that your sweat and urine take on a distinct odor of maple. Rarely, mothers taking fenugreek report having diarrhea, but it quickly subsides when the fenugreek is stopped. There have also been reports of some asthmatic women developing symptoms while taking fenugreek.

Blessed thistle is also helpful in stimulating milk production. Like fenugreek, this herb is available in capsule form. The typical dosage is three capsules (390 milligrams per capsule) three times a day. Blessed thistle and fenugreek can be safely used together.

9. Consider using a pharmaceutical drug to augment your milk production. Metoclopramide (Reglan) is available in the United States primarily for gastric reflux. Although the U.S. Food and Drug Administration has not approved it for the purpose of stimulating milk production, several studies have shown the drug to be effective and safe for increasing milk supplies. The typical dosage is 10 milligrams every 6 to 8 hours for 14 days. Metoclopramide has not been shown to cause any problems for a nursing baby—in fact, it is occasionally prescribed for infants. It may, however, make the mother sleepy. More worrisome side effects, such as agitation, are uncommon; when they occur, the drug should be discontinued. If taken longer than a few weeks, metoclopramide can lead to depression that may not resolve by simply discontinuing the medication. It should therefore not be taken for more than two courses.

Another drug that has come into favor for increasing milk production is domperidone (Motilium). It apparently works by stimulating the pituitary gland to produce more prolactin, the hormone that stimulates the breast to produce milk. The typical dosage is 20 milligrams four times per day, although some professionals recommend starting with 10 milligrams four times per day for the first week.

Although domperidone is marketed only as a treatment for disorders of the gastrointestinal tract, several studies show that it safely increases milk production, and the American Academy of Pediatrics has approved the drug (as well as metoclopramide) as safe to take while nursing. Because domperidone does not enter the brain tissue in significant amounts, it has far less frequent side effects than metoclopramide. Possible side effects in the mother—headache, abdominal cramps, and dry mouth—are extremely uncommon. Very little of the medication enters the breast milk—less, in fact, than the amount babies are given directly as treatment for gastric reflux. (At this writing, the U.S. Food and Drug Administration has just issued a warning about domperidone, because of several reports of sickness after the drug was administered in high intravenous doses, as treatment for gastrointestinal disturbances. According to Thomas Hale, a professor of pediatrics and pharmacology at Texas Tech University School of Medicine, this use of the drug caused blood levels 80 to 150 times higher than that of nursing women who take domperidone orally in normal doses.)

Domperidone is available in most countries of the world. Although it is not manufactured in the United States, it can be made here by special compounding pharmacies. But it is much less expensive, and available without a prescription, through Vanuatu in New Zealand (see Appendix A, page 246).

10. Find a supplemental feeding method that suits you. Many lactation professionals, fearing bottle feeding would interfere with the baby's ability at the breast, suggest using a nursing supplementer (see Appendix A, page 245), a cup, a soft tube, a finger, or an eye dropper. If one of these methods is recommended to you and it works well, terrific. But if you find it too frustrating or time consuming, use a bottle. After the first few days of breastfeeding, supplementing by bottle rarely causes "nipple confusion."

11. Weigh your baby every few days to make sure that she is gaining well. After each weighing, re-estimate her milk needs, because as she gains weight her milk needs will increase. Two hours after your last pumping, express your milk instead of nursing, then re-estimate your milk production. Hopefully it will also have increased, so that you can decrease or even eliminate any formula supplementation.

12. Once your baby is gaining well, her nursing seems more vigorous, and you are supplementing nursings only with your breast milk, you might try eliminating some of the supplement. For a few days, offer the baby only half of the milk that you are expressing, and freeze the rest. If the baby gains well over these few days, continue pumping, but don't offer her any of the expressed milk. If the baby continues to gain an ounce a day without any supplement, gradually stop pumping. Continue to have your baby weighed weekly.

If treatment fails. Although the technique just outlined will normally reverse a case of underfeeding right away, sometimes, when breast engorgement has been severe and little milk has been removed during this critical period, the decline in milk production can be difficult to reverse. In unusual instances, a mother fails to produce enough milk. This sometimes happens to women who have had breast surgery, particularly if the surgical incision was made around the areola (see "Nursing after Breast Surgery," page 86). Other women who cannot produce milk are those with insufficient glandular (milk-producing) tissue, or "hypoplastic" breasts (see page 40).

In any of these situations, lack of support from family, friends, and health professionals can only make matters worse. But even with all of the best information and support, things sometimes don't turn out as we hope. If after giving breastfeeding your best effort you end up having to bottle-feed, you have not failed as a mother. Be proud of your efforts to nurse, and concentrate on providing your baby with all of the cuddling and loving that you can. Detailed information about formula and bottle feeding can be found in *The Nursing Mother's Guide to Weaning* (see "Suggested Supplemental Reading," page 298).

Some mothers with insufficient milk production have found that continuing to nurse with a nursing supplementer has been a rewarding experience. Others have found nursing supplementers to be cumbersome and frustrating. Another option, particularly if the baby has become frustrated at the breast, is to bottle-feed and then nurse. "Comfort nursing"—nursing just after bottle feedings, in between bottle feedings, or during the night—may be a pleasant experience for both mother and baby.

3 SPECIAL MOTHERS, SPECIAL BABIES

Nursing can be a special challenge in certain circumstances—situations that may result from a longstanding condition or that may take you completely by surprise. Either way, you may be tempted to give up the idea of breastfeeding altogether. The specific guidelines in this chapter should help you make a realistic appraisal of your situation and find, I hope, the happiest solution for you and your baby.

SPECIAL MOTHERS

MEDICAL REASONS FOR
NOT BREASTFEEDING

Although most medical conditions a mother might have pose no harm to her nursing infant, a few are reasons to delay or even forego breastfeeding.

A mother with active tuberculosis should not breastfeed—or have any physical contact with her baby—until treatment has been administered for one to three weeks, after which she can no longer transmit the infection. During this period, she can express her milk to maintain her supply, but she should discard the milk she expresses. Afterward she can safely be reunited with her infant, and she can breastfeed.

A woman with hepatitis can generally breastfeed safely. If she has viral hepatitis, also known as infectious hepatitis or hepatitis A, her baby should be immunized with gamma globulin. If she has an active case of hepatitis B or persistent hepatitis B surface antigen (HBsAg), her baby should receive hepatitis B–specific immunoglobulin (HBIG) immediately after delivery. She can begin breastfeeding as soon as the shot is given, but her baby should also receive the first in a series of hepatitis B vaccines within 24 hours of birth. For women with hepatitis C, the Centers for Disease Control and Prevention, the American Academy of Pediatrics, and the National Institutes of Health support breastfeeding. Although it is theoretically possible to transmit hepatitis C to a baby through breastfeeding, several research studies have shown that breastfeeding does not increase the risk of transmission. A nursing mother may be more likely to infect her baby, though, if—

- She herself develops the disease in late pregnancy, and therefore doesn't develop antibodies before she begins breastfeeding;
- She has an active hepatitis infection with a high level of the virus in her blood while she is nursing; or
- Her nipples bleed.

Mothers with the human immunodeficiency virus (HIV) are discouraged from breastfeeding until more is known about transmission of the virus.

A woman infected with cytomegalovirus (CMV) can safely breastfeed her baby if he was born at full term. If the baby was born prematurely, he may be CMV-negative; that is, he may not have received antibodies against the disease during pregnancy and so may be vulnerable to the infection. The virus can be destroyed, however, by freezing the breast milk at 0 degrees Fahrenheit for at least three days.

A mother with herpes simplex, in the form of either cold sores on or near the mouth or genital lesions, can nurse her baby. It is important, however, that anyone with a herpes sore take certain precautions in handling a baby to avoid transmitting the infection. (See "The Mother with Herpes," page 97.)

Breastfeeding is also safe when a woman is infected with toxoplasmosis.

A mother infected with Lyme disease should be immediately treated, and so should her baby. The mother can breastfeed if she has begun antibiotic treatment and her baby is healthy.

Because human T-cell leukemia virus type 1 (HTLV-1) can be transmitted through breast milk, a woman infected with this virus should forego breastfeeding. (HTLV-1 is rare in North America, but it is increasingly common in other parts of the world. It is associated with the development of leukemia and lymphoma.)

A woman who develops chicken pox within the six days before delivery should be isolated from her baby, although someone else can feed the baby the mother's expressed milk. The mother and baby can be reunited after she becomes noninfectious, typically after seven days.

Although the overwhelming majority of women can produce a full supply of milk for their infants, even after a setback due to infrequent nursing or inadequate sucking (see pages 68 to 75), a few mothers are unable to produce enough milk. A low milk supply can occur when a mother has had extensive breast surgery (see "Nursing after Breast Surgery," page 86). A relatively uncommon condition is that of insufficient glandular tissue, or hypoplasia. In this case a mother finds that her breasts did not enlarge during pregnancy and did not undergo any changes (such as becoming heavier or fuller or leaking milk) during the first week after delivery. Most often the mother has widely spaced breasts; one may be significantly smaller than the other. She can still nurse her baby by using a nursing supplementation device designed to provide the extra milk needed (see page 245).

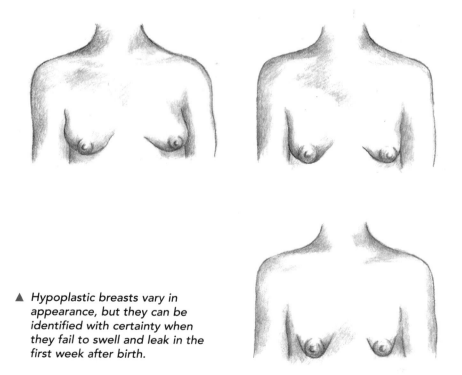

▲ *Hypoplastic breasts vary in appearance, but they can be identified with certainty when they fail to swell and leak in the first week after birth.*

Nursing after Breast Surgery

When performed prior to a woman's giving birth, minor breast surgery such as a biopsy or removal of a lump seldom affects the woman's ability to nurse unless the incision was made on the nipple or areola. A woman who has undergone a mastectomy can nurse on the remaining breast, and by nursing frequently she may be able to provide most or all of the milk that her baby needs. A breast that has been subject to radiation therapy produces little or no milk, but, again, the other breast should produce milk normally.

When a surgical implantation has been performed to alter the size and shape of the breasts, milk production is usually not affected unless the milk ducts have been severed (this may be the case if the incision was made along the edge of the areola). In the case of a breast reduction, milk production depends on the extensiveness of the surgery. When the nipples have been relocated on the breasts, some or all of the ducts have usually been severed, and so the milk supply is often threatened.

When a mother's milk ducts may have been severed, her baby should be observed closely for signs of low milk intake. I recommend a weight check by three to four days of age and every couple of days thereafter. A weight loss of 10 percent or more, or failure to gain an ounce a day after five days of age, indicates a baby needs supplemental feedings.

If you have had breast surgery involving an incision around the areola, you may benefit from renting a fully automatic electric breast pump and using it starting on the third day post partum. Pump for five minutes on each breast right after each daytime and evening nursing; pump both breasts at once, if possible. This can help in bringing in a more plentiful milk supply. For further guidance, see "Underfeeding and Weight Loss," page 76.

Recently I've worked with several women who have had breast reduction surgery yet have successfully brought in a full supply of milk. For some of these women, using an electric pump after each nursing helped a great deal in building an initially low milk supply. Some of the mothers found that using a nursing supplementation device (see page 245) helped to increase production as well. In all of these cases, however, two to eight weeks' effort was required before milk production totally met the baby's milk needs.

When the milk supply is clearly insufficient and shows no signs of increasing, a mother can still continue breastfeeding indefinitely, if she wishes. A nursing supplementation device may help to keep the baby from preferring the bottle.

NURSING AN ADOPTED BABY

More and more mothers who are planning to adopt babies are considering breastfeeding them. An infant's suck can stimulate milk production whether or not the mother has ever had or nursed a baby before, and even if she has reached menopause. Most adoptive mothers, however, need to supplement their breast milk, many for the entire time they are nursing. Probably the safest and most convenient way to supplement breastfeeding is with a nursing supplementation device, which is specifically designed for this situation (see Appendix A, page 245, for ordering information).

Some women's enthusiastic claims of producing abundant milk for their adopted babies may set up other adoptive mothers for disappointment. It is impossible to predict whether an adoptive mother will be able to produce milk, or how much she will produce, even if she is currently nursing or has recently nursed another baby. Adoptive nursing will be most successful if you focus on the relationship between you and your baby, rather than on milk production. Measure your success by whether the experience truly helps make the baby yours.

Before the baby arrives, it is wise to learn as much as possible about breastfeeding and adoptive nursing. Be sure to talk with a pediatrician who will be supportive of your efforts. A lactation professional may be able to refer you to other adoptive mothers who have nursed their babies.

▶ *As the baby nurses, she can get immediate satisfaction through a supplementation device.*

Nursing an adoptive baby doesn't require any advance preparation; you can simply put the baby to the breast and see what happens. In this case, though, you may or may not eventually produce significant amounts of breast milk. But if you know at least several weeks in advance that your baby is coming, you may be able to increase your chance of producing ample milk by following one of the protocols, or treatment plans, developed by Jack Newman, a physician, and Lenore Goldfarb, a lactation professional. These protocols are described below.

When your baby arrives, he may be easily persuaded to begin nursing, or he may require a great deal of patience and persistence. In general, the younger the baby is, the easier the transition from the bottle to the breast will be. See page 69 for assistance in getting the baby to nurse.

Most adoptive mothers need to supplement their milk with formula. Some women try to increase their milk production by using formula in only minimal amounts or by overdiluting it. But these practices often result in stressed, underfed babies.

If you've decided to use a supplementation device, you may be hoping for donations of breast milk to use in it, and perhaps you've already received offers of donated milk. But don't expect others to continue donations indefinitely. It can be a real effort for nursing mothers to collect extra milk. There is also a possibility that infectious diseases, including HIV and hepatitis, could be transmitted through donated milk.

Women who have breastfed adopted children often say that it has been one of the most memorable and rewarding experiences of their lives. You may especially enjoy nursing your adopted baby when she is older and you needn't concern yourself so much about milk production. Moments spent soothing a tired, hurt, or frustrated baby or toddler at the breast are priceless for any nursing mother.

The Newman-Goldfarb protocols

These regimens have helped over five hundred adoptive mothers, relactating mothers, and "intended" mothers (those who have used surrogates to carry a baby to term) to bring in substantial milk supplies. Each protocol involves pumping, preferably with a fully automatic pump and a double-pump kit, and taking both a birth-control pill, to hormonally mimic pregnancy, and a *galactogogue*, a medication that stimulates milk production. There are three protocols: a regular one, an accelerated one, and a third just for postmenopausal women. As a rule, the longer you follow your protocol, the more milk you will produce. If you're fertile, you'll need to use an alternative form of contraception while following the protocol.

The protocols described here are designed to mimic what happens before and after pregnancy. During pregnancy a woman's body produces increasing amounts of progesterone, estrogen, and lactogen, via the placenta, and prolactin, via the pituitary gland. These hormones ready the breasts for breastfeeding. Once pregnancy is completed, progesterone and estrogen levels drop and prolactin levels increase, resulting in lactation.

Birth-control pills can provide the estrogen and progesterone needed to simulate pregnancy (they do not supply prolactin or lactogen). To induce lactation, you will need to take monophasic birth-control pills—that is, all active ones, with no sugar pills—every day, without breaks. Each pill should contain at least .035 milligram ethinyl estradiol (estrogen) and at least 1.0 milligram norethindrone or an equivalent progestin. Acceptable birth-control pills include Ortho Novum 1/35, Necon 1/35, Demulen 1/35, Norethin 1/35E, Norinyl 1+35, Zovia 1/35, and Yasmin.

Women who have a history of thrombosis, cardiac condition, or severe hypertension shouldn't take birth-control pills, and other women can't tolerate their side effects. Several women have tried estrogen patches, estrogen lotion, or progesterone cream instead. If you have mild hypertension, you may be able to reduce it enough by taking methyldopa (Aldomet) to make birth-control pills safe for you. Methyldopa has the added benefit of increasing milk supply, and it is approved by the American Academy of Pediatrics for use in breastfeeding mothers.

Since birth-control pills sometimes cause depression, women with a history of depression generally don't take them. But several such women have followed the protocols while taking the antidepressant sertraline (Zoloft), which studies show to be safe during breastfeeding.

The galactologue that should be taken along with the birth-control pill is domperidone (Motilium). Although domperidone is marketed only for disorders of the gastrointestinal tract, it also stimulates milk production. Domperidone has few side effects (compared with metaclopramide, especially; see "Underfeeding and Weight Loss" on page 76), and it can be ordered inexpensively and without a prescription through a pharmacy in Vanuatu (see Appendix A, page 246). For best absorption, take domperidone a half-hour before meals.

Adoptive nursing mothers may need to take domperidone for the entire time they are nursing. Fortunately, side effects from domperidone are rare even when it is taken for many months. For more information about this drug, see "Treatment Measures for Underfeeding," pages 79–80, and Appendix A, page 246.

Consult your doctor before beginning to follow one of the protocols. If your doctor is not familiar with the process of inducing lactation, find an experienced lactation professional who is. See Appendix A, page 240, for help in locating one, or ask if one is available at the hospital or birthing center where the baby will be born. If you use a lactation professional, be sure your physician knows that you plan to breastfeed and receives a copy of the protocol.

The regular protocol. This plan is suitable for an intended mother (one expecting a baby via surrogacy) or for an adoptive mother with a long lead time. Women who follow this protocol are generally able to meet most if not all of their babies' needs for milk until the babies are weaned.

1. At least six months before the baby is due, take an active birth-control pill daily and 10 milligrams domperidone four times per day for one week.

2. After a week, increase the domperidone dosage to 20 milligrams four times per day, and continue taking the birth-control pill. Your breasts will swell, although the birth-control pill will actually suppress milk production, as happens during pregnancy. Don't pump or take any milk-augmenting herbs.

3. Six weeks before the baby is due, stop taking the birth-control pill, but continue taking 20 milligrams domperidone four times a day. You should experience vaginal bleeding; if you don't, you may need an exam to find out if you're pregnant.

    Begin pumping your breasts, every three hours if possible during the day, and at least once at night. Pump 5 to 7 minutes on the low or medium setting, and then massage, stroke, and rapidly shake both breasts.

    Stopping the birth-control pill while continuing to take domperidone and beginning to pump your breasts should cause a rapid decrease in the level of progesterone in your blood and a rapid increase in the level of prolactin. By mimicking what happens after pregnancy and birth, this process should cause your milk to come in.

    Once you have started pumping, you can also take some dietary measures to augment your milk supply. Three times a day, with meals, take three capsules each of blessed thistle

(390 milligrams per capsule) and fenugreek (610 milligrams per capsule). For more information on these herbal supplements, see "Treatment Measures for Underfeeding" on page 77. Try also to eat oatmeal at least three times a week, since women on the protocols have noticed significant increases in their milk supplies when they eat oatmeal regularly. You should also drink water whenever you are thirsty and avoid caffeine.

Your milk may come in over just a few days, or it may take a week or two; everyone responds differently. The milk will first appear as clear drops, which will gradually become an opaque white. Then the milk will begin begin to spray while you pump, and finally to flow in a steady stream. Save the milk for your baby (see "Collecting and Storing Your Milk," page 186).

4. When the baby arrives, nurse as soon as possible. Nurse the baby often, whenever he seems hungry or at least eight times in 24 hours. Supplement your milk as necessary with formula or donated milk, fed by bottle or through a nursing supplementation device (see "Underfeeding and Weight Loss," page 76). Until you have an ample milk supply, it's a good idea to pump for 10 minutes after each feeding.

    Continue taking domperidone—20 milligrams four times per day—and fenugreek and blessed thistle until your milk supply is well established. Once you have an ample milk supply, you may be able to decrease the domperidone and even eliminate it completely. To avoid dramatic drops in your milk supply, however, you should decrease the dose very slowly, by one pill per day.

The accelerated protocol. This plan is suitable for intended mothers (those expecting babies through surrogacy) or adoptive mothers who have only two to six months to prepare.

1. Take an active combination birth-control pill for 30 to 60 days nonstop along with 20 milligrams of domperidone four times a day. The best birth-control pill for the accelerated protocol is Yasmin, since it contains 3 milligrams of progesterone; the other combination pills contain only 1 milligram (the estrogen content is the same in Yasmin and the other pills). Many women have found that breast changes—enlargement by one cup size and the onset of a heavy, full, tender feeling—occur more rapidly with Yasmin than with

other birth-control pills. Expect that the rapid start of medications will cause fatigue.

2. If breast changes occur within 30 days, stop taking the birth-
    control pill but continue taking domperidone. Otherwise,
    continue taking both medications until your breasts swell.
    Then begin pumping as in the regular protocol, with a fully
    automatic pump and a double-pump kit, and taking the
    dietary measures described for the regular protocol. Store as
    much breast milk as you can (see "Collecting and Storing
    Your Milk," page 186).

3. When you begin nursing, continue taking domperidone.
    Nurse the baby often, whenever he seems hungry or at least
    eight times in 24 hours. Until you have an ample milk
    supply, it's a good idea to pump for 10 minutes after each
    feeding. Supplement your milk as necessary with formula
    or donated milk, fed by bottle or through a nursing supple-
    mentation device (see "Underfeeding and Weight Loss,"
    page 76).

The menopausal protocol. If you've reached menopause naturally
or had your reproductive organs surgically removed, you can still
bring in a milk supply and breastfeed. All you need are breasts and a
functioning pituitary gland.

1. If you're undergoing hormone-replacement therapy, stop.
    Instead, take an active combination birth-control pill once a
    day. The birth-control pill will provide enough estrogen and
    progesterone to keep your menopausal symptoms at bay
    while also readying your breasts for milk production.
    Because of its higher progesterone content, the best birth-
    control pill for the menopausal protocol is Yasmin. For the
    first week, you should also take 10 milligrams domperidone
    four times a day.

2. After the first week, increase the domperidone dosage to 20
    milligrams four times a day, and continue to take a daily
    birth-control pill. You'll need to take both medications for at
    least 60 days and until your breasts swell by one cup size
    and begin to feel full, heavy, and tender.

3. When you've experienced these breast changes and have
    taken both the birth-control pill and the full dosage of dom-
    peridone for at least 60 days, begin pumping your breasts,
    following the guidelines for the regular protocol. Take the
    dietary measures described for the regular protocol, too.

4. If your menopausal symptoms resume, you can reduce them by consuming soy products, especially soy milk and soy butter, which contain phytoestrogens. Consume only as much soy as you need to stop your hot flashes; too much would decrease your milk supply.

Deciding whether to use a protocol The decision whether or not to follow a Newman-Goldfarb protocol may depend on how much time you have. The regular protocol might increase your milk supply more than other measures would, but only if you can follow the regimen for six months or more. This may be easy if you're using a surrogate mother, in which case you'll know about the pregnancy from the beginning. If you're adopting internationally, also, you may learn about your baby several months before you bring the baby home. But sometimes a baby's homecoming is postponed, for as long as two months or even longer. A baby four months old or older who has been regularly bottle-fed is likely to refuse the breast. He may be persuaded, but if you don't want to go to great lengths to do so you may not want to take on the protocol.

Many adoptive parents don't know until weeks or just days in advance that they can bring their baby home. Sadly, the earlier in the pregnancy that an adoptive family is told they have been matched with a baby, the more likely it is that the birth mother will change her plans. Many women start the protocol in anticipation of adopting and then end up with no baby to nurse, or they continue pumping month after month with no news of the baby. Even those who are able to pump an impressive amount of milk find they cannot bear to keep up the pumping indefinitely.

For every mother who follows the regular protocol, brings in a good milk supply, and then acquires a baby to nurse within a reasonable amount of time, several others run into problems. Side-effects can be quite a concern. Some women on the protocols experience weight gain, depression and tearfulness, exhaustion, swelling of the legs, and extremely sore and swollen breasts. Some mothers follow the protocol for four months or longer and still don't get a full milk supply. After such an investment of time and energy, this is a great disappointment. In contrast, quite a few women get full milk supplies from taking domperidone alone while nursing or pumping, and others do so with just breast stimulation and herbs.

The accelerated protocol is recommended for women who have one to two months to prepare, and also for those who expect to get a baby in just weeks or days or who are already nursing. When used for less than 60 days, this protocol has not proven more effective than other methods of stimulating milk production. Some lactation consultants feel that mothers who have less than 60 days to prepare will get a milk supply established faster by pumping and taking domperidone without birth-control pills, which suppress milk production as long as they are taken and for several weeks afterward.

A potential risk for women who use the protocols is coming to see a nursing supplementer as evidence of failure, rather than as an the important tool it is for both nurturing a baby and stimulating milk production. When a mother with a low milk supply nurses as much as possible, using a supplementer as needed, her supply often increases. More importantly, she establishes a long-term nursing relationship with her baby, which is beneficial in so many ways.

RELACTATION

For a variety of reasons, a mother may want to begin nursing after initially starting her baby on the bottle, or to resume nursing after weaning her baby.

In general, the less time that has elapsed since weaning, the more likely bringing back a full milk supply will be. A mother with a five-day-old baby who has never nursed, or a six-week-old who has been weaned for just a few days, should be able to bring in a full milk supply within several days. After longer periods without nursing or expressing milk, the ability to re-establish full milk production will vary from woman to woman.

Always critical to milk production is frequent and regular stimulation and emptying of the breasts. This means that either a vigorous nursing baby or a fully automatic electric breast pump should be draining both breasts at least every two and a half hours during the day and evening and twice at night. Even when a baby is willing to nurse, using a fully automatic pump with a double-pump kit for 5 to 10 minutes right after nursing can be very helpful in collecting any residual milk the baby leaves behind and stimulating further milk production.

The herb fenugreek is also very helpful in stimulating increased milk production. You can make tea from fenugreek seeds, but more effective are the concentrated capsules sold in health-food stores. If you take two to three capsules three times a day, you should notice an increase in milk supply within one to three days. For more information, see "Treatment Measures for Underfeeding," page 77.

Two pharmaceutical drugs have been used to stimulate milk production, metoclopramide (Reglan) and domperidone (Motilium). The usual dose of metoclopramide is 10 milligrams every six to eight hours for 10 to 14 days. Women usually notice increased breast fullness 48 to 72 hours after starting on the drug. The medication works best with frequent breast stimulation and emptying, and is most effective during the first 12 weeks post partum. If no change is observed after five days, the medication probably will not be helpful. Although some mothers find a second two-week course helpful, I would discourage longer use of metoclopramide, which often causes depression when used for long periods.

The other drug used to stimulate milk production, domperidone, works like metoclopramide, has fewer side effects, and can be ordered without a prescription through a pharmacy in Vanuatu. The typical dose is 20 milligrams four times per day.

For more information on metaclopramide and domperidone, see "Treatment Measures for Underfeeding," page 77. For information on ordering domperidone, see Appendix A, page 246.

Regardless of the time that has elapsed between weaning and attempting relactation, a baby will need supplemental feedings until full milk production has been established. You could continue bottle feeding, but offer the bottle only after nursing and give slightly less formula than before. Or you could use a nursing supplementation device, which would allow you to feed your baby the supplement while he sucks at the breast. This option may be most helpful if your baby acts frustrated while nursing. See page 245 for information on nursing supplementation devices.

Knowing how much supplemental milk and formula to give a baby can be a bit of a guessing game. If you have a fully automatic breast pump, you can use the method described in "Underfeeding and Weight Loss" on page 76 to estimate your milk production and your baby's supplemental milk needs. Without this type of pump, you will need to rely solely on weight checks.

Whether or not you're using an automatic pump, have your baby weighed every day or two during the first week or so after you start trying to relactate. Until your baby is three or four months old, he should gain an ounce a day. Gaining less than this amount indicates that he needs more supplemental milk or formula; gaining more may mean that the supplement should be cut back a little. Always weigh your baby naked, on the same scale, at about the same time of day, and just before a feeding.

Recently, a very accurate electronic baby scale for home use has become available for rent. This scale can also be used before and after feedings to determine how much milk the baby takes from the breast. See Appendix A, page 247, for information on renting a scale.

THE DIABETIC MOTHER

Many diabetic mothers enjoy the advantages of nursing. For them breastfeeding often stimulates a remission-like response, resulting in a decreased need for insulin and an increased need for calories. Babies of diabetic mothers are less likely to develop the disease themselves later in life if they are breastfed rather than formula-fed.

If you are diabetic, your requirements for insulin and calories will need to be closely monitored—especially during the early hours after delivery, when your insulin needs will drop dramatically.

For the first day or two, your newborn's blood sugar must be closely watched as her body adjusts to receiving less glucose than it did during pregnancy. She may need frequent nursing, and possibly supplemental glucose by nipple or IV, until her glucose levels stabilize. Because the infant of the diabetic mother is commonly delivered a few weeks early, she may also have respiratory problems, and she is more prone to becoming jaundiced.

Throughout the months of breastfeeding, careful monitoring of your glucose level, insulin dose, and caloric requirements must continue. As the baby stimulates increased milk production, you and your doctor will need to adjust your insulin dosage and caloric intake to prevent insulin reactions.

You should take particular care to avoid sore nipples and breast infections. This means giving careful attention to correct positioning of the baby, watching for signs of thrush (yeast) in the baby's mouth and on the nipples (see pages 53–55), and getting plenty of rest. Yeast infections are very common in the diabetic mother and her infant. Plugged ducts and other early signs of breast infection (see pages 140–144) should be treated promptly.

When weaning begins and milk production declines, you'll need to readjust your insulin dosage and diet again. This will be easier if you wean the baby slowly.

THE MOTHER WITH HERPES

If you have an active genital herpes lesion or a positive culture near your due date, and you therefore deliver by cesarean, you will most likely be given a private hospital room. So long as the lesion is well covered and you wash your hands thoroughly before feedings, you can nurse the baby safely without gloves. There is no reason that you cannot share a room with the baby as long as you maintain these basic precautions. Should you have a herpes outbreak at home, the same principles apply.

Herpes Type I lesions are generally those that develop above the waist, usually on the mouth. Frequently they appear as cold sores or fever blisters. It is important for you, or any other person with an active lesion, to wash your hands thoroughly before touching the baby, and, of course, to avoid placing her in contact with the sores.

Occasionally a mother will develop a herpes lesion on her breast, nipple, or areola. Should you have such an outbreak, express your milk until the lesion is gone.

THE EPILEPTIC MOTHER

Most medications to control the occurrence of epileptic seizures are considered safe for nursing; however, it is best to check out any drug with your doctor. Major anticonvulsant medications are listed in Appendix C, where their safety is discussed.

A nursing mother with epilepsy offers these suggestions for others (Brewster, 1979):

- Have cribs or playpens available in various areas of the house; place gates across stairways and doorways.

- Nurse in a large upholstered chair, or pad the arms of a rocking chair.

- Use guard rails and pillows around the bed for night nursing.

- When alone on outings with the baby, tag the stroller or carrier with the name of the baby and the name of a person to contact in the event that you have a seizure.

Nursing and Thyroid Conditions

Hypothyroidism

Symptoms of an underactive thyroid gland may include extreme fatigue, poor appetite, and sometimes a low milk supply. Thyroid replacement quickly reverses these symptoms. The mother who is taking medication for hypothyroidism can breastfeed, as these drugs do not affect the baby.

Hyperthyroidism

Occasionally a doctor will discover that a nursing mother has an enlarged thyroid gland. Signs of hyperthyroidism include weight loss, increased appetite, nervousness, rapid heart rate, and palpitations. Nursing must be discontinued for at least 48 hours when radioactive iodine is used for diagnostic testing; however, other tests are available that do not require this interruption. If radioactive iodine is used, express or pump your milk and dispose of it.

If you are taking medication for an overactive thyroid gland, you can breastfeed as long as the specific medication is considered safe for the nursing baby. PTU (propylthiouracil) is the drug of choice, since it has the least effect on a baby's thyroid gland. The baby's thyroid level should be monitored by a pediatrician.

Pumping Exclusively

For any of a variety of reasons, a woman may find herself pumping all of her baby's milk and feeding it by bottle instead of nursing. It may be that the baby has not been able to latch on to the breast or, in some cases, that the mother actually prefers to feed her baby this way. Many women who have exclusively pumped have managed to produce enough milk to meet their babies' needs for months or even a year or beyond.

Pumping full time for a baby requires a great deal of dedication and discipline. Unlike a baby, a pump does not signal for attention, and for most women pumping is more a chore than a pleasure. To feed your baby entirely or mostly on your own milk, however, is to give him an extra-special gift.

Frequent and effective pumping during the first week after birth is critical in establishing an abundant milk supply. After a week of infrequent or ineffective pumping, it is much more difficult to increase low production.

Effective pumping requires a high-quality, comfortable pump. Starting out with a hospital-grade fully automatic pump is the very best way to bring in a full milk supply—about 24 ounces per day during the first month after birth. A double-pump kit, which collects milk from both breasts at once, makes pumping quicker and usually more effective in establishing and maintaining milk production.

Since hospital-grade pumps are expensive, most women who use them rent them rather than buy them. If your income is low or modest, you may qualify for a rent-free automatic pump through the WIC program (see page 241). In any case, long-term pump rental is much less costly than buying formula.

It is essential to pump often—every two to three hours during the day and at least once in the night, or at least eight times in each 24 hours. You must also spend enough time at each pumping to drain both breasts completely, since it is the frequent, thorough drainage of the breasts that signals them to increase milk production and keep it high. Some women can completely drain the breasts by pumping for 10 minutes or less, but others need a longer time. Until you're sure how much time you need, pump until the milk stops flowing and then a couple of minutes longer.

Pumping shouldn't hurt. Initially, you may be more comfortable if you apply a thin coat of lanolin around the base of the nipples before starting to pump (for sources of modified, nonallergenic lanolin, see Appendix A, page 247). If pumping is painful even with lanolin, it may be that the breast shield doesn't fit right.

A properly fitting breast shield allows for pulling and releasing of the nipple without causing the nipple to swell against the sides of the tunnel. If the nipples swell too much in the tunnel, the breast won't drain completely. To find out if the shield opening is too small, pump 20 minutes after a previous pumping. If you get more than $1/2$ ounce at the second pumping, the shield may be preventing the breast from draining completely. If you're using a Medela or Ameda automatic pump, you can order a collection kit with a large or extra-large shield from the manufacturer (see Appendix A, page 243); your hospital or lactation professional might be able to provide one, too.

Once a generous milk supply is established—at least 24 ounces per day—some women invest in their own near-hospital-grade pump, such as Medela's Pump in Style or Hollister's Purely Yours (see pages 176–185 for more information about pumps). Other mothers, however, are unable to maintain high production with these newer pumps and continue to require a hospital-grade model.

After the first month, some women are able to maintain their production level with seven pumpings each 24 hours. With less frequent pumping than this, however, most women find that their supply often drops below the baby's needs. A few women are blessed with massive production. If you are one of these, you can freeze the extra milk for later use—for feeding directly or mixing with cereal.

You milk supply will need to grow as your baby does. From the fifth day after birth until about four months, babies generally gain about an ounce per day. After four months of age, their weight gain typically slows to about a half ounce per day. This means that they require about 20 to 24 ounces of milk per day in the first month and then their intake gradually increases to about 36 ounces per day by the beginning of the fourth month. Their intake stays at about that level until other foods slowly begin to replace breast milk in the diet.

Bottle-fed babies often drink more than they need for normal growth, even when they're fed breast milk rather than formula. Since overfeeding a baby can lead to obesity later, you may want to keep track of how much milk your baby is taking. These guidelines may be helpful: During the first month, offer about 1 ounce per hour, or 3 ounces every two and a half to three hours. After the first month, offer up to $1\frac{1}{2}$ ounces per hour, or $4\frac{1}{2}$ ounces every three hours. If your baby seems to want more milk than this, try to keep in mind that babies often fuss when they are overstimulated, tired, or uncomfortable. A breastfeeding mother may put her baby to the breast hourly when he is tired or cranky, but he doesn't get a large meal at each comfort feeding. Carrying your baby or offering a pacifier between feedings may help in calming him. (If your baby is very fussy, see "Fussiness, Colic, and Reflux," pages 152–162.)

Some women who exclusively pump do struggle with low milk production. If your production is lower than suggested here, you can take measures to increase it.

1. Be sure that you are not pregnant or using estrogen-containing birth control. Although health-care providers may tell you otherwise, combination birth-control pills and the vaginal ring with estrogen typically lessen milk production. The progesterone-only "mini-pill" is usually fine.

2. Be sure you are using a hospital-grade pump and double-pump kit.

3. To be sure your pump is working efficiently, give it a checkup. Check the tubing, connections, and white rubber diaphragms. If the diaphragms get small tears, the pump will not work efficiently.

4. Pump *at least* eight times a day—more if you can manage. During the night, pump at least every four hours. Since your body produces more prolactin at night, pumping then has a strong influence on production.

5. If your pump offers a speed option, pump so that the nipple is pulled and released about 50 times a minute. Pumping too slow or too fast can affect the volume of milk expressed.

6. Consider taking fenugreek capsules. See "Underfeeding and Weight Loss," page 76 or "Relactation," page 94.

7. Instead of or along with fenugreek, try the herb blessed thistle, which also helps to stimulate milk production. For more information on blessed thistle, see "Underfeeding and Weight Loss," page 79.

If you're pumping out of necessity rather than choice, it may be helpful to know that many babies become able and willing to take the breast despite months of bottle feeding. If your baby has been unable to latch on and suck well, it is still worthwhile to try nursing periodically. A lactation professional may be able to help you.

Special Babies

Medical Reasons for Not Breastfeeding

Infants born with galactosemia, a rare inherited disorder, lack the enzyme necessary to break down the sugar found in all milk, including breast milk. They must be fed a special lactose-free formula.

Infants with phenylketonuria (PKU), another rare metabolic disorder, require a diet with little phenylalanine, an amino acid. Because breast milk is low in phenylalanine, a baby with PKU may be breast-fed part time provided she is also fed phenylalanine-free formula. Her blood level of phenylalanine must be monitored to be sure that it remains between 5 and 10 milligrams per deciliter.

The Premature Baby

The days after giving birth to a premature baby can be overwhelming, particularly if the baby is sick or very immature. The mother of a premie may have doubts about many things, including her ability to nurse the baby.

If your baby is born prematurely, it is especially important that he receive your milk. Your milk is particularly suited for his special growth needs and is easier for him to digest than formula. Premature infants are at greater risk for developing infections and are less able to cope with them when they arise. The antibodies in your milk will provide your baby with protection against many of these infections. Your milk may also reduce your premature baby's risk of developing cerebral palsy (Lucas, 1992). By providing breast milk, many mothers of premature infants have felt that they were able to contribute something special to their baby's well-being.

If your baby is three to five weeks early, you may be able to begin breastfeeding right away. The sick or very small premie may be unable to nurse for a while, but you can express your milk for him until he is well or mature enough to begin nursing. In this way he can still receive your milk, and you will have established your milk supply by the time he is ready to begin breastfeeding.

Nursing the baby born three to five weeks early Usually babies who are born a few weeks before their due date are encouraged to begin breastfeeding within the first hours or days of birth. Barring any health complications, most physicians and nurses treat these babies like other newborns and encourage parents to do the same.

Generally, babies who are born a few weeks too soon tend to be rather sleepy; they may or may not start out as vigorous nursers. Many fall asleep at the breast before they have had an adequate feeding. For this reason, they often fail to gain weight. A few days of a baby's sluggish nursing and limited milk removal can also have a devastating effect on milk production.

An effective preventive measure is the use of a fully automatic electric breast pump. Starting on the third day post partum, a mother should pump for five minutes on each breast right after each daytime and evening nursing. This ensures an abundant milk supply for the baby even if his sucking is sluggish. The residual milk collected can be frozen for later use.

The baby should be watched closely for the reassuring signs of adequate milk intake. She should be weighed at 10 to 12 days, or sooner if suspicions arise that she may not be taking enough milk. If the baby is back to her birth weight at 10 to 12 days, the pumping can be gradually discontinued over a few days. Weighing the baby once again before returning the pump to the rental station will give further reassurance that nursing is going well, providing the baby has gained an ounce a day since the tenth day.

If the baby loses 10 percent or more of her birth weight, she should be offered the residual milk being collected.

Expressing milk for your baby   If your baby is unable to nurse, start expressing your colostrum as soon after delivery as possible. Colostrum is especially beneficial for him because it is highly concentrated with protective antibodies. The nursing staff should provide you with a suitable pump and instructions for collecting and storing your milk. Most maternity units have an electric breast pump available. A fully automatic electric breast pump is most suited for a mother who is pumping around the clock for a premie. (See page 243 for information on electric breast pump rentals.) If your baby is being transferred to another hospital for care, ask the transport team about their procedures for collecting, storing, and transporting your milk. If you will be following the baby to a special care nursery in another city, try to get a pump to take along with you.

You may receive differing bits of advice on how often and how long to pump your breasts. Keep in mind that your supply of milk depends on the frequent stimulation of your breasts. You should plan on expressing milk as often as your baby would nurse, or at least eight times in 24 hours. Many nursery staffs suggest that women pump every three to four hours during the day and sleep all night. With this limited stimulation, most mothers find that after a while their milk supplies dwindle. Determine a reasonable schedule for yourself that includes eight pumpings in 24 hours. Some mothers prefer to express their milk every three hours around the clock, whereas others would rather pump more often during the day so they can sleep for longer periods at night.

When you first begin to express milk you will probably start out getting just a few drops of colostrum. Until your milk is in, pump each breast for about five minutes, then return to each breast a second time for a few more minutes.

After your milk is in, pump each breast until the flow subsides. Return to each breast a second or third time for a few more minutes. Gently massaging each breast for a minute or so before you begin and while you are pumping will help your milk to let down. The whole process should take no more than 20 to 30 minutes. If you can get a double-pump kit, pump for 10 to 15 minutes. Double-pumping not only decreases the time needed to pump but maximizes milk production.

Ideally, you should pump more milk than your baby requires. Building and maintaining a volume of at least 24 ounces per day will allow you to have extra milk on reserve should you experience a temporary decline (due to stress or illness, for example) during your baby's hospitalization. Having an abundant supply will also help your baby get milk more easily once she is able to nurse.

Take special care when expressing and storing your milk. Wash your hands before handling your breasts or any of the pump equipment. All pump parts that come in contact with the milk or your breasts must be thoroughly scrubbed with hot soapy water after each use and sterilized in boiling water or a dishwasher twice a day. Your daily bath or shower will cleanse your breasts sufficiently.

After collecting your milk, pour it into a sterile container of the nursery staff's preference. To avoid wasting milk, ask your baby's nurses how much to put in each container. Milk cannot be refrozen or refrigerated after it has been thawed or warmed; whatever is left over after the feeding must be thrown out.

Whenever possible, provide freshly expressed or refrigerated milk for your baby. Freezing the milk preserves many, but not all, of its protective substances. You can keep your milk for 24 to 48 hours in the refrigerator or for up to three months in the freezer.

When transporting your refrigerated or frozen milk to the hospital, pack the containers in ice inside a small ice chest or cooler. Some families use refreezable ice packs to keep the milk cold, or, if they're traveling a long distance, dry ice to keep the milk frozen.

Be sure to let the hospital staff know about any medications you take, including any over-the-counter medicines, such as pain relievers or cold remedies. Although most medications are safe to take while nursing, a few could harm a sick or premature infant.

Expressing milk longer than two weeks. Depending on your baby's maturity and general progress, you may find yourself expressing milk for a while. It is important that you eat well, get plenty to drink, and rest enough to maintain your own energy as well as your milk supply.

If you notice that your milk supply is declining a few days in a row, you will need to assess the situation and make whatever adjustments are necessary. The most common cause of a decreasing milk supply is infrequent expression—fewer than eight times in 24 hours. Although a few mothers can maintain a good milk supply expressing less often than this, most are not able to keep up their supply after a few weeks. If you have been using a hand pump, rent an electric pump. Most mothers find an electric pump requires less effort and is more efficient as well as convenient.

Besides increasing the number of pumpings per day, switch from one breast to the other as soon as you notice the flow slowing down; do this several times during each feeding. This technique is very effective for increasing milk production. Pumping both breasts simultaneously, using one of the double-pump kits manufactured by the makers of electric breast pumps, is also a very effective way to increase your milk production and decrease your pumping time. With these kits most mothers can express their milk in 10 to 15 minutes.

Occasionally you may notice that your milk supply drops when you and your baby have a difficult day. This is normal and usually temporary. Stress can temporarily decrease your milk supply. The following suggestions have proved helpful when this occurs:

- Pump regularly, every two to three hours.
- Take a short nap or a warm bath just before expressing.
- Apply moist heat to your breasts before expressing.
- Massage each breast as you are pumping, or stimulate the opposite nipple.
- Ask someone to rub your back between the shoulder blades while you are pumping.
- If possible, hold the baby while you are pumping at the hospital, or keep a photo of your baby with your pump.

Should you find that your are having a chronic problem with low milk production, see "Pumping Exclusively," page 98.

| **Supplementing breast milk** | Many premature infants need extra nutrients, such as calcium and phosphorus, in addition to breast milk. Although breast milk alone is |

the perfect food for a full-term infant, a premie's nutritional needs, because of her small size and immaturity, may be somewhat different. Commercially prepared fortifiers can be mixed with breast milk to provide for these special needs. Usually, the fortifiers are discontinued before the baby leaves the hospital.

Some premature babies need a more concentrated source of calories. If this is the case with your baby, ask about feeding hind milk. This is the fattier milk produced after the first few minutes of pumping. To collect hind milk separately from foremilk, pump for about two minutes after the milk lets down, then stop pumping and switch collection bottles. Pump again until the breast is completely drained. Label the first bottle as foremilk, the second as hind milk. Provide the hind milk for the baby's immediate needs, and freeze the foremilk for the future (for use during separations or for supplementation). Feeding hind milk for a week or two can be very helpful in achieving good weight gain in a premie.

| **When breastfeeding begins** | When the time arrives to begin nursing the premature infant, most mothers have very high expectations. Premies' abilities at the breast vary greatly, but most are unable to |

complete an entire feeding at first.

Have a nurse help you during the first few sessions. Your goal is to position the baby well for nursing and to encourage her to latch on to the breast. These early practice sessions go best when the baby is awake and alert and the breast is not overly full. Keeping the baby wrapped in a blanket may discourage her interest. A premie will usually stay warm undressed next to her mother's body. Lay a blanket over your shoulder and the baby to limit heat loss. The nurse can check the baby's skin temperature after five to ten minutes.

The cross-over hold and the football hold (see pages 31–34) are the positions of choice for nursing a premature baby. Both of these positions support the baby's head. Place your hand around the baby's head with your fingers behind and below her ears. Support her neck and shoulders with the palm of your hand and your wrist. With your

◀ *Getting a premie to latch on requires extra effort: Use the cross-over or football hold.*

thumb at the point where the baby's nose will touch the breast, compress the breast with your fingers. Lightly stroke the baby's upper lip with your nipple to signal her to open her mouth wide. As soon as she does, pull her head and shoulders toward you so that the nipple is on top of her tongue and far back in her mouth.

Again, premies' abilities at the breast vary greatly, so be patient. As long as you have positioned your baby correctly and are encouraging her to open her mouth, you have been successful.

Once latched on to the breast and sucking, a premie may fall asleep after just a few minutes. She may need a supplement after nursing until she is feeding more vigorously at the breast. Most hospitals give nursing premies supplements by bottle; others give them by passing a soft tube through the nose or mouth into the stomach, to avoid "nipple confusion."

While you are nursing your baby, you should be able to hear her swallowing. This means she is sucking effectively and getting your milk. If you do not hear swallowing, make sure the baby is actually latched on to the breast. Her suction should be so strong that it is hard to pull her off. You should not see dimples in her cheeks or hear clicking noises as she sucks. These signs would indicate she was sucking on her tongue and not on your breast.

When the baby seems interested in the second breast, you can simply pass her head and body over to the other side, or you can reposition her entirely in the opposite arm using the football hold.

To maintain your milk supply, be sure to pump after these feeding sessions with the baby. The collected milk can be used for supplemental feedings.

Difficult latch-on. Many premature infants have difficulty latching on, due to their own immaturity as well as having received rubber nipples as pacifiers or for feedings. Some babies have trouble learning to lower their tongue to latch on, whereas others seem unable to identify their mothers' nipples in their mouths.

If your baby has not been able to latch on to the breast, refer to "Difficult Latch-on: Refusal to Nurse," pages 68–73. In my experience, most premature infants learn to nurse after a period of daily practice sessions.

The transition to full-time nursing While you and the baby are establishing nursing, you may wonder how much milk the baby is taking. Although mothers and health professionals often try to gauge the baby's milk intake by how long he nurses, how much swallowing can be heard, or whether the baby will take supplemental milk, none of these methods are accurate. The best way to determine the baby's milk intake is to weigh him before and after nursing, in the same diaper and clothing, on an electronic gram scale. Each gram of weight gain equals 1 milliliter of milk intake. Recent studies have shown that these pre- and postfeeding weights are extremely accurate in indicating how much milk a baby has taken.

How much breast milk a baby should take at each feeding can be calculated by multiplying the baby's weight in kilograms by 22.5 (a pounds-to-kilogram conversion chart is in Appendix B, page 252). This will give you in milliliters the amount of milk a baby needs at each of eight daily feedings. For example, if a baby weighs 2.2 kilograms he will need 49.5, or approximately 50, milliliters of milk each time he nurses for a total of eight times per day. If the baby takes 30 milliliters during the nursing session, he will need an additional 20 milliliters after nursing to gain an adequate amount of weight.

While you are in the hospital, have your baby weighed on the nursery's scale before and after nursings. If you do this at each nursing, you should begin to develop a sense of how much milk the baby is taking at any feeding. Once at home, you may need weight checks only every two days or so to help you judge how much supplement the baby needs. If you want to continue pre- and postfeeding weight checks at home, rent a highly accurate electronic scale (see Appendix A, page 247).

Until your baby is nursing without any supplemental feedings, you will need to continue expressing milk after each nursing to maintain your milk supply.

NURSING MORE THAN ONE

Needless to say, caring for two or more babies takes a tremendous amount of time and energy. Breastfeeding multiples is not only more healthful and economical than giving them formula, but in many ways it is more convenient. Mothers of twins often say that nursing is easier and less time-consuming than preparing and feeding bottles, particularly when a woman has mastered the skill of nursing two babies at the same time.

Although many mothers worry about being able to produce enough milk for more than one baby, most women are capable of producing plenty of milk for two and even three babies.

As soon as you become aware of the twins during pregnancy, you should begin some special preparations. You will want to arrange for as much help as possible, of course, for the first several weeks after the birth. It's also a good idea to get to know other mothers who have successfully nursed their twins. Many communities have organizations for mothers of twins. You might also contact your local breastfeeding support group; such a group usually provides literature on caring for and nursing twins.

Approximately half of all twins are born prematurely. During pregnancy you can do much to lessen the risk of premature delivery and other complications by maintaining a diet high in calories—at least 2,900 a day—and protein—at least 110 grams a day. Talk with your health-care provider about monitoring yourself for signs of preterm labor.

Establishing an abundant milk supply
Making enough milk for two or more babies depends on the frequent and complete drainage of the breasts. Multiples who are born early or of low birth weight may not consistently nurse effectively enough to stimulate abundant milk production. For this reason I recommend using a fully automatic breast pump, with a double-pump kit, whenever multiples are born three or

more weeks before the due date or weigh less than six pounds each. Even if your babies are healthy and latching on to the breast frequently, pump for five to ten minutes after each nursing to ensure complete drainage of the breasts and to stimulate abundant milk production. Read "The Premature Baby," page 101, for more information on nursing premature babies and pumping after feedings.

If the babies are in a special-care nursery and are unable to nurse, use the electric pump at least eight times in every 24 hours. Be sure to review the information on expressing milk for your premie on page 103. You should aim to produce at least 16 ounces of milk per day for each of your babies.

Breastfeeding two or more

You should nurse each of your babies at least eight times in every 24 hours. This may mean waking smaller babies every three hours during the day and evening for feedings, and every four to five hours in the night, until they are gaining weight well without any supplementation.

▲ *You can nurse twins simultaneously using the cradle hold, the football hold, or a combination of the two.*

Some mothers prefer nursing their babies together as much as possible, whereas others choose to nurse them separately. Nursing two at once certainly saves time, and it may be necessary when both of the babies are hungry. If you want to nurse the babies together, there are three basic positions you can try:

- both babies in the cuddle hold with their legs side by side or crossed over each other,

- one baby in the cuddle hold and the other in the football hold, or

- both babies in the football hold.

During the early weeks, you may need assistance getting the babies on the breast at the same time. You will also probably need a few pillows for positioning. (A special pillow is available for nursing twins. See Appendix A, page 247, for ordering information.) It may be easier to position the baby who nurses less vigorously first, and then put the vigorous nurser to the breast. Nursing the twins simultaneously should get easier as they get older and need less head support and assistance latching on.

Nursing the babies separately, each baby on one breast only, may be easier to manage and will allow you more time with each individually. You may decide to feed each baby whenever she seems hungry or you may prefer to encourage the babies to eat and sleep on approximately the same schedule. To maintain a similar routine for both babies, simply offer the breast to the second baby, waking her if necessary, after nursing the first. Although most twins eventually develop a preference for one breast over the other, it is wise to alternate the babies at each feeding during the early weeks so the breasts will be evenly stimulated; this is particularly important when one baby is more active than the other. Keeping a simple written record may be helpful at first.

Mothers of triplets generally nurse two babies simultaneously and then the third baby from both breasts, or else another caregiver gives the third baby a bottle. Again, alternate the babies from one feeding to the next.

During the early weeks, if the babies are gaining weight adequately, substituting bottle feedings for nursings is best avoided. You want to be sure your breasts are stimulated by the babies' sucking so that milk production remains adequate. Foregoing the bottle also helps to minimize the occurrence of plugged ducts and breast infections.

Caring for yourself

For the mother who is nursing two or more babies, plenty of rest, food, and drink is essential. Most nursing mothers are naturally more hungry and thirsty than usual, but if you take on too much and become fatigued, you may lose your appetite and too much weight. Nutritionists recommend that a mother nursing twins consume at least 3,000 calories daily. Your diet should include high-protein foods and a quart or more of milk a day, the equivalent in other dairy products, or a calcium supplement. Vitamin C and B-complex supplements or brewer's yeast may also be beneficial.

THE BABY WITH A BIRTH DEFECT

It may be that the baby with a birth defect needs his mother's milk, and the comfort and security of the breast, even more than other infants. Nursing such a baby is usually possible, but it is important that the mother is supported in her efforts. Although some mothers of babies with birth defects have been discouraged from attempting breastfeeding, many have gone on to nurse their babies successfully.

Depending on your baby's problem, you may be able to begin nursing right after birth, or you may need to express milk for a while (see "Expressing Milk for Your Baby," page 103). Whatever the circumstances, it may be helpful to seek guidance from a lactation professional. Some helpful publications are listed at the end of the book.

Heart defect

Infants with heart defects generally have little trouble breastfeeding. The exception is the baby with a severe defect, who may become easily fatigued or stressed during feedings; he will start breathing rapidly, his heart will beat faster, and his overall color may change. His growth may be greatly affected due to the abnormality of his heart. He may also be more prone to infections, and therefore in greater need of breast milk than other babies.

The baby who becomes stressed during feedings needs to be nursed more frequently for shorter periods of time. He may also be more comfortable when held upright for nursing, as in the football hold.

Cleft lip and palate

The baby born with a cleft lip, palate, or both may have difficulty latching on and sucking effectively, so feeding her may present special challenges. Breastfeeding may be possible, depending on the location and extent of the cleft, but most of these babies, particularly those with cleft palates, are unable to get enough milk from nursing alone. Yet breast milk helps reduce the number and severity of ear and respiratory infections, which are more common in these babies than others. Many mothers, therefore, pump their milk and feed it to their babies with whatever method works best for the baby.

The baby born with a cleft lip alone may have little difficulty nursing. Until the lip is repaired, usually when the baby is several weeks old, she will need to be positioned with the cleft sealed, to permit suction. You may ensure a complete seal just by pulling the baby close against your breast, so that your breast occludes the cleft, or you may need to place your finger or thumb over the cleft. If you find that your baby has more difficulty nursing on one side than the other, try using the football hold on that side.

Whether a baby with a cleft palate can nurse usually depends on the location and extent of the cleft. When it is in the soft palate only, the baby may or may not be able to nurse without much difficulty. It's best to position her so her head is raised; milk may come out of her nose if she is fed while lying flat. Ask the baby's doctor or a lactation professional about techniques to help babies with cleft palates to breastfeed. An infant may be fitted with a plastic dental appliance, an obturator, that covers the cleft and allows for adequate sucking. Some lactation professionals have reported success with the use of a nursing supplementation device (see Appendix A, page 245) and certain positioning techniques.

If your baby has a cleft lip or palate, try to get her to latch on and suck as soon as possible after birth. If she can't latch on, use a fully automatic electric breast pump after every nursing, or every two to three hours around the clock, to stimulate and maintain an abundant milk supply. An electric breast pump, ideally a lightweight model with a double-pump collection kit, is most efficient and requires the least amount of pumping time.

Bottle-feeding a baby with a cleft lip or palate can also be challenging. The nursing staff should have special feeders of various types that you can try while you are in the hospital. The Haberman Feeder, a device for feeding babies with cleft palates, has worked well for some of my clients. See Appendix A, page 248, for ordering information.

When a baby has an extensive cleft palate or a cleft palate and lip, nursing can be difficult or even impossible. In this case you will probably need to express milk for some time. Although long-term pump rental is far cheaper than purchasing infant formula, you may eventually decide to use formula anyway, since a cleft palate is generally not repaired until the baby is one to two years old.

Whether your baby has a cleft lip, a cleft palate, or both, closely monitor her weight to make sure that she is getting enough to eat. If you are exclusively bottle-feeding, see Appendix B, pages 252–253, to determine how much milk she needs at each feeding. If your baby is able to latch on and suck, you may be unsure how effective she is at getting milk and whether she needs supplemental milk, or how much she needs, to gain weight. In this case, weigh the baby every couple of days, and adjust the amount of supplement according to how much she is gaining. Renting an electronic scale for a few weeks may be helpful. You can use the scale before and after nursings to determine how much milk the baby is getting, or use it simply to get an accurate daily weight. See Appendix A, page 247, to locate a scale.

DEVELOPMENTAL AND NEUROLOGICAL PROBLEMS

Babies with Down syndrome, hydrocephalus, spina bifida, and other neurological problems benefit greatly from breastfeeding. Because nursing provides frequent physical contact, it may be especially valuable to such a baby's development.

If the baby's sucking ability is affected, teaching him to nurse will require a great deal of patience. Professional guidance from a lactation professional experienced with such problems and a physical therapist may be necessary. When a baby is unable to suck, some mothers have been able to nurse with a nursing supplementation device (see page 245) or have provided their expressed milk in a bottle. Sources of additional information are listed at the end of the book.

Down syndrome   Not only will nursing further the development of the infant with Down syndrome, but it may also provide him with much needed protection from illness, as he is at greater risk than most babies for developing infections. Although many infants with Down syndrome are able to nurse, some have difficulty learning how to latch on and suck effectively. The baby may have weak muscle tone and may act sleepy and uninterested in the breast. He will need to be roused frequently for nursing (see "Sleepy Baby," page 63).

Typically, the baby with Down syndrome grows slowly. If his suck is weak and inefficient, you may need to pump out the milk he leaves in the breast. Regular pumping will allow you to maintain sufficient milk production and provide the baby extra milk, which you can feed as a supplement after each nursing.

Hydrocephalus and spina bifida These birth defects are usually corrected surgically as soon as possible. Until the baby can begin to nurse, the mother must express milk (see "Expressing Milk for Your Baby," page 103). For many such babies, positioning at the breast requires special attention so that they are protected and comfortable.

Cerebral palsy Babies with cerebral palsy may also be able to nurse, depending on the severity of their conditions. Breastfeeding problems that occur are usually related to either (1) poor muscle tone and a weak suck or (2) excessive muscle tone (rigidity and abnormal posture), tongue thrusting, clenching of the jaw, and difficulty swallowing. Both of these situations usually lead to slow weight gain. Some infants with cerebral palsy are able to breastfeed successfully with a nursing supplementation device. (See page 245 for more information on these devices.)

4 THE LEARNING PERIOD: THE FIRST TWO MONTHS

After the first week, you may already be feeling energetic and confident in your abilities as a new mother—or you may be exhausted, overwhelmed, and perhaps troubled with some aspect of breastfeeding. In any case, it is important to realize that the first two months after giving birth are a time for adjustment and learning. Mothers normally have questions and concerns about themselves, their babies, and nursing during this period.

Now That You Are Post Partum

Caring for Yourself

The postpartum period is the six weeks after birth in which all of the many changes of pregnancy are reversed. Virtually every system in your body will go through some readjustment. As your uterus shrinks in size and the inner lining is shed, a new layer is formed. The vaginal flow, or lochia, decreases in amount and progresses to pink or brown and then to white. Many women continue bleeding throughout the first month. Intermittent spotting is common. Too much activity may cause the lochia to become heavier and turn red again—a signal that you should slow down.

If you have had a vaginal birth, your vagina, perineum, urethra, and rectum have undergone considerable stress. Frequent warm baths will speed healing and help relieve discomfort—unless you have hemorrhoids, in which case ice packs may be preferable. Menstrual pads soaked with witch hazel and then frozen are very soothing for hemorrhoids.

Kegel's exercises will help this area return to normal by strengthening the entire pelvic floor. These exercises are simple and can be done anytime, anywhere. Several times a day, tightly squeeze the muscles around your anus, then around your vagina and urethra. Gradually work up to 100 "kegels" a day.

If you have had a cesarean birth, keep in mind you are recovering from major abdominal surgery. Most likely, you will need to take pain medication during the first week or so at home. You may perhaps be bothered by an uncomfortable feeling that your abdomen may fall out. A lightweight girdle can provide some welcome support.

Constipation is a common complaint after giving birth. It can best be prevented by drinking plenty of fluids, adding fiber to your diet, and getting regular exercise. Be aware that some laxatives could affect the baby through your milk, causing cramping, excessive stools, and even weight loss.

Night sweats are very common in the first few days after birth, and they sometimes continue for several weeks.

Most women experience emotional changes during the postpartum period. Anxiety, moodiness, and irritability are common responses to the hormonal changes that occur after giving birth, as well as to the tremendous responsibility of caring for a new baby. Some mothers notice other postpartum "symptoms" such as forgetfulness, inability to concentrate, and difficulty expressing thoughts. These problems seem to pass with time. If you fall prey, though, to exhaustion, poor nutrition, and isolation from other adults, depression may be the result.

Starting at approximately six to twelve weeks after birth, some women experience generalized hair loss *(telogeneffluvium)*. Because of the hormonal changes following birth, hair follicles simultaneously move from the growing phase (which they were in during pregnancy) to the resting phase of their development. Postpartum hair loss is seldom severe, and women never go bald because of it. The period of hair loss lasts about three to six months. It has no relationship to breastfeeding.

Because of the rapid physical changes of the postpartum period and the tremendous amount of time and energy needed to care for and nurse a baby, rest should continue to take high priority for all new mothers. Lack of rest can slow your recovery from the birth and may lead to tension, inability to cope, poor appetite, and depression. Be sure to take at least one nap every day during these important first weeks. Do essential household chores and activities while the baby is awake so that you can nap together. Tucking the baby in with you at nap time and bedtime may help you both sleep better. Getting plenty of rest now will contribute greatly to your sense of well-being and your breastfeeding success.

After a couple of weeks some light exercise can do much to renew your energy. A brisk twenty-minute walk with the baby can be invigorating; the fresh air will do you both good. Many community centers offer exercise programs for new mothers. Often the babies are included in the exercises, and sometimes infant care is provided. Despite recent claims that exercise causes lactic acid to build up in breast milk, and babies therefore to refuse to nurse, moderate exercise has little or no effect on the composition or volume of breast milk. With whatever activity you choose, however, you will want to start out slowly.

You may feel isolated as a new mother, especially if you have left work or school—and most of your friends—to care for the baby. You need adult companionship. Check with your childbirth educator or public-health nurse about groups for new mothers. Attending La Leche League meetings, taking a mother-baby exercise class, or socializing with women from your childbirth class are excellent ways of getting out with the baby and getting to know other new mothers.

▲ *New mothers' groups provide opportunities for socializing as well as learning about infant development.*

YOUR NUTRITIONAL NEEDS

Drinking enough

Maintaining an adequate intake of fluids is usually not a problem for the nursing mother. Most women are naturally more thirsty while they are breastfeeding. Contrary to popular belief, forcing fluids beyond satisfying natural thirst does not increase milk production. But when a nursing mother does not drink at least six to eight glasses of fluids every day, dark, concentrated urine and constipation usually result. She may need to make a conscious effort to increase her fluid intake.

Eating well

Provided you established good eating habits during pregnancy and gained an adequate amount of weight, you probably won't need to change your diet much at all. Nursing mothers are often told to add about five hundred calories, including 65 grams of protein, to their pre-pregnancy diets. Recent research, however, indicates that many mothers may not need this much food, so don't feel you must eat more than you want. You can get extra nutrients in between-meal snacks, perhaps during nursings: half a sandwich and a glass of milk, three glasses of juice, or one-half cup of shelled peanuts will supply about five hundred calories. Some mothers experience a temporary

◀ *Don't expect to be able to get into your jeans for several weeks, at least.*

loss of appetite during the first couple of weeks after delivery. Eating smaller, more frequent meals or snacks may be more appealing than three big meals each day.

You may feel discouraged that your shape is not back to normal. The clothes in your closet may seem as if they belonged to someone else. Although you lost some weight when you delivered, you are probably still pounds away from your usual weight. During the early months of breastfeeding, this extra fat is a useful energy store. If you let your appetite guide you as you continue nursing, you will probably lose the excess weight gradually and feel good while doing it. Dieting during the early weeks is not a good idea.

If you like, you can estimate your daily caloric needs by multiplying your current weight by 15. Add 500 to your total to meet the caloric needs of nursing (if you are nursing twins, add 1,000 calories).

$$
\begin{array}{rl}
Example: & 135 \text{ pounds} \\
& \times\ 15 \\
\hline
& 2{,}025 \text{ calories} \\
& +\ 500 \text{ calories} \\
\hline
& 2{,}525 \text{ calories}
\end{array}
$$

If you are a moderately active woman, you can expect to lose a pound every two to three weeks on this diet. If you are very active and have no problem controlling your weight, or if you burn calories slowly, you will need to adjust the figures somewhat: multiply your weight by 17 (high activity) or 13 (low activity). The minimal safe food intake for a nursing mother of average size is about 1,800 calories per day.

Low-carbohydrate diets are not recommended while nursing. Whole grains and other high-carbohydrate foods supply nursing mothers with vitamins, minerals, and energy. Low-carbohydrate diets are dehydrating, and they often cause constipation, fatigue, and sleeping problems.

Milk production is largely independent of nutritional intake during the first few months of breastfeeding. This is partly because the fat accumulated in pregnancy is available as a ready supply of calories. When a mother's diet is inadequate, however, milk production usually continues at her expense—leading to fatigue, listlessness, and rapid weight loss.

Some women have trouble finding time to fix nutritious meals for themselves when they are at home alone with the baby. If you find yourself in this situation, start the day with a good breakfast, and then snack throughout the day on nutritious foods such as hard-boiled eggs, leftover chicken or beef, cheese, peanut butter, yogurt, seeds, and nuts. Don't forget the fiber: whole-wheat bread, whole-grain crackers, and fruits and raw vegetables will provide it. Some mothers have developed their own favorite recipes for high-energy blender drinks using ingredients such as milk, yogurt, nuts, and bananas or other fruits.

Avoid snacking on foods or drinks that are high in sugar. Refined sugar provides only "empty" calories—empty, that is, of vitamins and minerals. Soda, cookies, and candy will not provide sustaining energy and may diminish your desire for more nutritious foods.

Mothers who are vegetarians can certainly maintain a diet to support their nutritional needs. But since vitamin B_{12} is found only in the animal kingdom, deficiencies may occur when a mother maintains a "vegan" diet, excluding eggs and milk products as well as meat. Supplementation with up to 4 milligrams of vitamin B_{12} per day is recommended.

Although most nutritionists recommend that a nursing mother drink three 8-ounce glasses of milk a day, there is no need to drink milk if you don't like it or can't tolerate it. A woman's bone density tends to decrease somewhat during lactation even when her calcium intake is relatively high. This causes no long-term harm. The bones grow denser again after weaning, and some studies suggest that women who breastfeed actually reduce their risk of developing osteoporosis later in life.

Still, nutritionists recommend that breastfeeding women consume 1,000 milligrams of calcium per day. If you don't drink milk, make sure you're getting enough calcium from other sources, such as those listed in the table below.

Serving	Milligrams calcium
yogurt (8 oz.)	288
cheeses (1 oz. cheddar or swiss)	222
cottage cheese (½ cup)	110
tofu (½ cup)	68
corn tortilla (1)	42

Although dark green vegetables in general are rich in calcium (100 milligrams per half cup), the calcium they provide is poorly absorbed by the body. Broccoli is the one exception to this rule. If you do not use dairy products at all, then, calcium supplements may be necessary. The least expensive supplement, with the highest concentration of calcium, is calcium carbonate. Avoid bone meal and dolomite, as some types have been found to be contaminated with lead.

Dietary supplements

If you are well nourished, vitamin supplements are unnecessary while you are nursing, although you may need iron supplements if you are anemic after birth. Also, some nursing mothers develop vitamin B deficiencies, experiencing depression, irritability, impaired concentration, loss of appetite, and tingling or burning feet. A daily B-complex supplement is often prescribed to reverse these symptoms.

Sometimes nursing mothers are advised to take brewer's yeast, a natural source of B vitamins, iron, and protein. Some mothers feel it improves their milk supply or increases their overall energy level. Health-food stores carry brewer's yeast in a powdered form that can be mixed with juice or milk.

If you decide to take vitamin supplements or brewer's yeast, remember that they are no substitute for a varied diet of nutritious foods, and in large quantities they can sometimes be dangerous. There have been reports of fussiness in babies whose mothers take brewer's yeast or large doses of vitamin C. Vitamin B_6 supplements in large doses have been reported to reduce milk production.

Foods and other substances you may be wondering about

There are no foods that should be routinely avoided by nursing mothers, but occasionally a baby will be bothered by something the mother has eaten. Some babies fuss for up to 24 hours after their mothers have eaten garlic, onions, cabbage, broccoli, brussels sprouts, cauliflower, chiles, or beans. Citrus fruits and their juices, chocolate, and spices such as chili powder, curry powder, and cinnamon can also bother young nursing babies. If your baby has unusual and persistent symptoms such as sudden refusal to nurse, vomiting, diarrhea or green stools, gassiness, redness around the anus, fussiness at the breast, or colic symptoms, see "Concerns about the Baby," page 149.

Caffeine taken by the mother has been known to cause irritability and colic symptoms in some babies. Caffeine is present in coffee, tea, and many soft drinks. You may want to limit your intake of these beverages.

An occasional glass of wine or beer is not believed to harm a nursing infant. Because alcohol passes through the breast milk, however, moderation is essential.

Mothers who smoke have lower levels of vitamin C in their milk than nonsmokers. Breathing cigarette fumes increases a baby's risk of contracting bronchitis and pneumonia, and perhaps of succumbing to crib death. If you smoke, try to limit the amount, and don't do it around the baby.

NURSING YOUR BABY

YOUR NURSING STYLE

During the early weeks, each mother develops her own style of nursing. Many women feel comfortable putting their babies to breast whenever they signal the desire to nurse. Others expect their babies to fall into a predictable feeding schedule. They may be troubled when their babies nurse irregularly or want to nurse again soon after being fed. These mothers may worry that perhaps they have too little milk or that it is somehow inadequate. Sometimes they feel they must hold the baby off until a certain number of hours have passed since the last feeding. But the breasts do not need to rest for any period of time to build up a supply for the next feeding; they produce milk constantly. The expectation that a baby should nurse on some type of a schedule usually leads to frustration for both mother and baby—and not uncommonly to breastfeeding failure.

The typical newborn infant nurses between eight and twelve times in a 24-hour period, or about every one to three hours. Because of the ease with which breast milk is digested, nursing infants have been described as continuous feeders. Not only must a baby nurse often to satisfy her hunger and stimulate an adequate milk supply, but she also seeks out the breast to satisfy her needs for sucking, security, and comforting.

It is a common misconception that the breast empties in a certain number of minutes, and that a baby should be taken from the breast after those minutes have elapsed. In fact, most mothers experience the release of milk several times during a feeding. The length of time required to complete a feeding varies from baby to baby. The "all-business" nurser, who swallows continuously with few pauses, may be done in ten minutes, whereas the "dawdler" may take up to 45 minutes. The length of nursing time may vary in the same baby from feeding to feeding. Before long, most mothers can tell when their babies have had enough.

Some babies nurse from only one breast at a feeding some or most of the time. This is fine so long as the baby seems satisfied and is gaining weight adequately. You may prefer to offer only one breast per feeding, in fact, if you have an abundant milk supply. Your baby is more likely to drain the breast completely this way, and complete drainage helps prevent plugged milk ducts and breast infections. Your baby will also be sure to get the rich hind milk, which is produced only as a feeding comes to a close.

I strongly recommend that your baby be weighed at 10 to 14 days of age. Although many infants are not scheduled for a routine well-baby exam until three to four weeks of age, a weight check at two weeks can be very beneficial. If the baby is back to her birth weight or beyond, you can be reassured early on that your nursing relationship is progressing well. On the contrary, if the baby has not yet regained her birth weight, you can usually correct this quite easily. When a poor weight gain is not discovered until three or four weeks, it is more likely to upset everyone and may be harder to correct than it would have been at two weeks.

You may find that nursing is the most enjoyable part of your day—a time to sit back, relax, and simply enjoy being with your baby. But it may be difficult at times for you to break away from what you are doing or sit still long enough for the baby to have a leisurely nursing. It may help to make a special little nursing area for yourself—or two or three nooks in different parts of the house. You might want to include a book, some magazines, or a note pad within reach. Having the phone nearby may also be handy. Some mothers make a point of getting a snack or something to drink just before sitting down to nurse.

Many babies seem to get hungry whenever food is served. If you usually find yourself nursing while trying to eat dinner, you may find a baby swing handy. Some parents have found that taking the baby for a walk just before dinner lulls her to sleep so that they can eat without interruption.

YOUR MILK SUPPLY

During these early weeks your milk production may seem somewhat erratic. At times your breasts may feel as if they are bursting with milk. At other times you may worry that there is not enough milk, especially if your breasts seem empty and your baby wants to nurse all the time. Many mothers notice this happening around two to three weeks and then again at six weeks, when a baby normally experiences appetite spurts and nurses more often to stimulate increased milk production. You can expect fluctuations in your milk supply as production becomes regulated according to the baby's demands.

By six to eight weeks after birth, many mothers notice that their breasts seem smaller or feel less full. This does not usually mean that less milk is being produced, but only that the breasts are adjusting to the large amount of milk within and the baby's feeding pattern.

Some mothers misinterpret their babies' increased demands and their own softer breasts, and begin offering supplemental bottles. For most mothers and babies, this marks the beginning of the end of breastfeeding. The mother begins to assume that she cannot make enough milk for her baby, and she offers more and more formula instead of allowing the baby to increase her own supply of milk. After receiving formula the baby sleeps longer and nurses less often. He becomes increasingly frustrated at the breast as his mother's milk supply dwindles. For these mothers and babies, breastfeeding is soon over.

Some mothers try to satisfy their babies' hunger with solid foods. Introducing solids during these early weeks is also inappropriate, since young infants are both physiologically and developmentally unable to manage them. Their digestive systems and kidneys are not mature enough to handle cereals and other baby foods. Infants may develop allergies to solid foods given during this period because their immune systems are still immature.

Fluctuations in the fullness of your breasts and in your milk supply will probably pass by the end of the second month. In the meantime, you can be reassured that your milk supply is probably fine if you are nursing at least eight times in each 24-hour period and letting the baby suck for as long as he wants. If you are worried about your milk supply, though, have your baby weighed. A weight gain of at least an ounce a day will tell you that your baby is getting plenty to eat. If you have additional concerns about your milk supply, see "Underfeeding," page 162.

SCHEDULED FEEDINGS

In recent years, some parenting books and classes have promoted a philosophy of scheduled breastfeeding. Called Parent Directed Feeding, the program teaches parents to feed babies on a rigid three- to four-hour schedule and to eliminate nighttime feedings at an early age. The purpose is to relieve parental anxiety and instill a sense of order and discipline in the infant. Although most parents like the idea of predictable, widely spaced nursings and full nights of sleep from the early weeks on, these practices are often associated with low milk production, poor weight gain in the baby, and early weaning. Some babies subjected to this method have become dangerously thin and dehydrated.

Babies do best if they are nursed when they seem hungry. Parent Directed Feeding fails to take into account two important facts about breast milk and breastfeeding. First, nature has designed breast milk to be taken frequently. Low in protein, it is easily and quickly digested. Second, a mother's milk supply depends on frequent, complete drainage of the breasts. If she nurses fewer than seven times in a 24-hour period, her milk production generally declines. Although some mothers can meet their babies' needs with fewer than seven daily feedings, most cannot.

The American Academy of Pediatrics, and every other organization that supports breastfeeding, recommends that babies be fed whenever they show signs of hunger.

INFANT DIETARY SUPPLEMENTS

Vitamins

Because of recent reports of rickets among American infants, the American Academy of Pediatrics (AAP) now recommends that all children, including babies who are exclusively breastfed, consume at least 200 International Units of vitamin D per day beginning no later than two months after birth and continuing through childhood and adolescence. Since all infant formulas, like commercially produced cow's milk, are fortified with vitamin D, babies fed at least 500 milliliters (17.6 ounces) of formula daily get as much vitamin D as the AAP recommends. For exclusively breastfed babies, vitamin D is available in an over-the-counter liquid supplement, Tri-Vi-Sol, which also contains vitamins A and C. Cod liver oil, a supplement much hated by children of generations past, also contains vitamins A and D.

Rickets is a bone-softening disease most commonly caused by insufficient exposure to sunlight. Sunlight, not food additives or supplements, is "the biologically normal and most common way for humans of all ages to develop adequate levels of the hormone 'vitamin D,'" according to Cynthia Good Mojab, a research associate at La Leche League International. The amount of sunlight exposure needed to prevent vitamin D deficiency depends on such factors as latitude, season, altitude, weather, time of day, and air pollution. It also depends on how much skin is exposed, whether sunscreen is applied (since sunscreen prevents vitamin D production), and skin pigmentation. Virtually all recent cases of rickets have occurred in dark-skinned babies.

These cases of rickets are probably due in part to parents' over-reaction to warnings about skin cancer. All humans, babies and adults alike, need to spend time in the sun. The question of how much time was explored in a study of white, exclusively breastfed babies under six months of age in Cincinnati, Ohio. The babies achieved adequate vitamin D levels when exposed to sunlight for 30 minutes per week while wearing only a diaper (or four to five minutes a day, on average) or for two hours per week while fully clothed without a hat (or about 17 minutes a day, on average). Infants living further north than Cincinnati, which is situated at latitude 39° N, may need more sun exposure than this; infants living closer to the equator may need less. Dark-skinned infants may need more sun exposure than light-skinned infants, but researchers have yet to ascertain this. For all babies, the sun exposure must be direct; sunlight that has passed through windowpane glass, Plexiglas, or almost any other plastic does not allow the body to produce vitamin D because these materials absorb ultraviolet B radiation.

Experts agree that vitamin D supplementation is important for infants at risk of a deficiency—because they are rarely taken outdoors, because they are kept covered with clothing or sunscreen, or because they live at high latitudes. But the idea of giving supplemental vitamin D to all breastfed babies is quite controversial. According to Cynthia Good Mojab, no one has investigated the potential risks of vitamin D supplementation, such as aspiration of the supplement, harmful changes in the baby's gut, or increased susceptibility to infection. Since vitamin D is available in the United States only in combination with other vitamins, studies must include the risks of supplementing those vitamins, too.

If you want to avoid giving your baby vitamin D supplementation, you have several choices. While you're pregnant, you can get plenty of sunshine yourself; this will ensure that your baby is born with enough vitamin D stores to last two months even if she is never exposed to the sun. You can supplement the vitamin D your body makes with that available in a few foods naturally (salmon, sardines, herring, and eggs) and in others through "fortification" (especially milk). After your baby is two months old, you can maintain her vitamin D level by giving her some time in the sun most days. If you're not sure she is getting enough exposure to sunlight, you can ask your doctor to measure the level of vitamin D in her blood to determine whether supplementation is warranted.

Iron

The full-term newborn has sufficient stores of iron for the first six months after birth. The small amounts of iron in breast milk are very well utilized by the nursing infant, so iron supplementation is unnecessary. Furthermore, iron supplements can interfere with the protective properties of breast milk. The premature infant, however, is likely to use up her iron stores earlier than the full-term infant. Supplemental iron is recommended for the premature infant beginning at two months of age or earlier.

Fluoride

Fluoride given from infancy is believed to reduce cavities 50 to 65 percent during childhood. Even though a mother may drink fluoridated water, little fluoride reaches the baby through the breast milk. The American Academy of Pediatrics therefore recommends that a baby receive fluoride supplements of 0.25 milligram per day, unless she is being fed formula mixed with fluoridated water.

Some authorities, however, believe fluoride supplementation is unnecessary for the breastfed infant, and point out that too much fluoride can cause spotting of the tooth enamel. Additionally, some infants are reported to become fussy and irritable and to have gastrointestinal upsets after being given fluoride.

For these reasons, the American Academy of Pediatrics now recommends delaying fluoride supplements until a baby is six months old. Fluoride is available by prescription, either alone or in combination with vitamins A, C, and D (which most breastfed infants do not require).

LIFE WITH YOUR BABY

SLEEPING WITH YOUR BABY

Although mothers and babies have slept together at least as long as mammals have roamed the earth, recent warnings about the dangers of bed-sharing are worrying new parents. The American Academy of Pediatrics has stated that bed sharing can be hazardous under certain conditions, and in 1999 the Consumer Product Safety Commission recommended against parents and babies sleeping together at all. But many physicians, scientists, parents, and SIDS researchers—including one of the safety commissioners—disagree with the commission's recommendations.

Anthropological and developmental studies suggest that mothers and infants are biologically and psychologically designed to sleep next to each other. Parents who sleep with their infants report that they enjoy this closeness and find it makes nighttime parenting easier. Being close to the baby in the night means being more aware of her cues and therefore more responsive to her needs. Even though bed-sharing mothers and babies wake more frequently, they go back to sleep sooner and so get more sleep overall than mothers and babies who sleep separately. Babies who sleep with their parents also cry significantly less than babies who sleep alone.

Because bed-sharing mothers nurse more frequently, they produce more milk than they would otherwise. This can be especially important to women who must spend time apart from their babies during the day. Women who work outside the home also often find that bed sharing helps them feel more connected to their infants.

Dr. James McKenna, an expert on infant sleep, believes that a parent's close breathing may help regulate an infant's own breathing pattern, and that bed sharing may thus reduce instances of death from sleep apnea, or Sudden Infant Death Syndrome (SIDS). His review of studies suggests that when a mother and her baby are close enough during nighttime sleep to sense each other in at least two of four ways—sight, scent, sound, and touch—the baby's risk of succumbing to Sudden Infant Death Syndrome (SIDS) is significantly decreased. Dr. McKenna points out that the largest increases in bed sharing, in the United States and abroad, have occurred among middle-class whites, the very group that has experienced the sharpest declines in rates of SIDS and other infant deaths.

In his sleep laboratory at the University of Notre Dame, Dr. McKenna has found that bed-sharing mothers and their infants are extremely sensitive to each other's movements and physical condition throughout the night, across all sleep stages. For instance, healthy, full-term babies whose air passages become blocked alert their bed-sharing mothers and, under normal circumstances, maneuver out of danger. Babies who sleep alone, Dr. McKenna has found, spend more time in deeper stages of sleep, which may be harmful for those babies with inherent arousal deficiencies.

Other researchers have suggested that babies who sleep with their mothers develop into children who are independent, sociable, confident, and well able to handle stress. Children who have never slept in their parents' bed, say the researchers, are harder to control (according to their parents), less happy, and more prone to tantrums. Children who have always slept alone, moreover, are rated more fearful and more dependent on their parents than children who have always slept in their parents' beds.

There are certainly hazards to avoid in bed sharing, but there are hazards in laying the baby to sleep anywhere. Wherever the baby sleeps, the dangers are mostly the same: pillows, toys, and quilts that could suffocate; cords and ties that could strangle; gaps in which a baby could become wedged; heights from which she could fall; and overheating, which increases the risk of SIDS. Bed sharing poses the additional risk of overlying, but this is generally only a concern when other children are sleeping in the same bed or a parent is intoxicated or extremely exhausted. Generally, adults have a sense of their own boundaries even when asleep; this is why you don't fall out of bed at night.

For most of the benefits of bed sharing with no risk of overlying, you might try placing your baby's bed very close to your own. You can even buy a baby bed, a "co-sleeper," that attaches to an adult bed, so you can reach your baby without getting up even though she sleeps on a separate surface (see Appendix A, pages 248–249).

Following are some guidelines for safe infant sleep, with the parent or in a separate bed:

- Use a firm mattress that fits the bed or crib frame well, without gaps in which a baby could become wedged.

- Stretch the sheet tightly around the mattress.

- Avoid night clothes with strings or ties, both for the baby and, if you're sharing the bed, for yourself and your partner.

- Keep the baby's face uncovered.

- Leave off the bed pillows, comforters, feather beds, stuffed animals, lamb skins, and other soft things that could pose a risk of suffocation.

- Put the baby on her back or side to sleep. Babies sleeping face up are less likely to become victims of SIDS.

- Don't smoke, and don't let other people smoke in the house. Exposure to tobacco, both during pregnancy and during infancy, is associated with a higher risk of SIDS.

- Avoid overheating the room in which the baby sleeps, and avoid overdressing the baby.

- Avoid laying the baby to sleep near dangling cords or sashes.

- Don't leave a young baby, especially one born prematurely, to sleep in a car seat or infant seat. If the baby's upper body is inadequately supported, her airway may become blocked.

If your baby sleeps in a crib—

- Make sure the rails are no further than $2^3/8$ inches apart.
- Use a crib bumper with at least six ties. The ties should be no longer than 6 inches long.
- Hang any crib mobile well out of the baby's reach, and remove it when the baby starts to sit or reaches five months of age, whichever comes first.
- When the baby learns to sit, lower the mattress so that she can't fall out or climb over the side rail.
- When she learns to stand, set the mattress at its lowest level and remove any crib bumpers.
- When she reaches a height of 35 inches or the side rail is less than three-quarters of her height, move her to another bed.
- Remove any crib gym when a baby can get up on all fours.
- Dress the baby in a blanket sleeper instead of using a blanket. If you do use a blanket, make sure the baby's head remains uncovered.

If your baby sleeps with you—

- Don't leave the baby to sleep alone in your bed.
- Fasten back your hair, if it is very long.
- After drinking or taking drugs that may cause you to sleep too soundly, and at any time that you are extremely exhausted, put the baby to sleep in a separate bed.
- If your bed has head- or footboard railings, they should be spaced no wider than $2^3/8$ inches apart.
- Don't use bed rails in the baby's first year, since she could become wedged between the mattress and the side rail.
- Don't let an older sibling share a bed with an infant less than one year old.
- Don't share a waterbed with your baby, since the surface could hamper breathing if your baby were to turn face down.
- Don't place the bed against the wall or against other furniture, since the baby could become trapped in between.
- Don't sleep with the baby on a sofa or overstuffed chair.

ILLNESSES: YOURS AND THE BABY'S

When you come down with a minor illness such as a cold or flu, you need not interrupt breastfeeding. Most likely your baby will have already been exposed to the virus that caused you to get sick. In fact, the antibodies you produce against the illness will reach the baby through the milk and may protect him from getting the same sickness. Even though you may not feel much like eating, try to drink extra fluids to keep from getting dehydrated. Should you need to take a medication, even an over-the-counter drug, be sure to check on its safety for the baby (see Appendix C, page 254).

Temporary weaning is also unnecessary if you suspect you have a case of food poisoning, provided your only symptoms are vomiting, diarrhea, or both.

Your milk supply may seem low during or just after an illness, but a few days of frequent nursing will usually bring milk production back to normal.

Should you require hospitalization or surgery, you can continue breastfeeding. If you know ahead of time that you'll need a hospital stay, you can pump and save milk for any time that you may be unavailable to your baby. You may be able to arrange that your baby stay with you, although the hospital will probably require that another adult be there to care for the baby. Ask if the hospital has a fully automatic breast pump for you to use when you cannot nurse; if not, arrange to bring one along, with a double-pump kit. The hospital may even have a lactation professional on staff who can assist with any breastfeeding problems that arise during your hospitalization.

You won't need to express and throw out milk contaminated by an anesthetic or pain medication. By the time you awaken from anesthesia, there will not be enough of the drug in your body to be a problem for your baby. Pain medications are also safe. If you take *The Nursing Mother's Companion* to the hospital with you, you can refer to Appendix C (page 254) for information on other medications.

When you are not able to nurse your baby, express your milk every two to three hours during the day and evening and as often during the night as you usually feed the baby. Ask the nurses to wake you as often as you need to pump. They should be able to refrigerate your milk in clean containers that you can take home to your baby.

Should your baby become ill, nursing should certainly continue. Breast milk is the best source of fluids and nourishment for recovery and nursing the best source of comfort. But sickness often changes a baby's nursing pattern. He may nurse more than usual, or he may lose interest in feeding.

Ear infections, sore throats, and fever blisters may make nursing painful for the baby. As long as he is nursing infrequently or is refusing to nurse, be sure to express your milk every couple of hours to keep up your supply. Colds and stuffy noses may make nursing difficult for him. Holding him upright while feeding, using a humidifier in the room, or administering saline nose drops and using a bulb syringe may make nursing more comfortable.

Fever is a sign of infection. During the first four months, a temperature above 99°F., if taken in the armpit, or 101°F., if taken rectally, should be reported to the baby's doctor. If, besides having an elevated temperature, the baby doesn't act like his usual self or he nurses poorly, he should be checked by your doctor. The severity of a fever does not always correspond with the seriousness of an illness; a high fever may appear with a minor infection and a low fever may accompany a serious infection. Because a fever may lead to dehydration, frequent nursing is very important.

Diarrhea in the breastfed baby, although less common and usually less severe than in the formula-fed baby, is characterized by frequent (12 or more per day), extremely loose or watery bowel movements. Often the stools are foul-smelling, and they may contain mucus or blood. Since babies lose a great deal of fluid with diarrhea, they can easily become dehydrated, making frequent nursing important. With its high water content, breast milk helps replace the lost fluids. Diarrhea generally improves within three to five days. Fever, infrequent feedings, or signs of dehydration (dry mouth, few wet diapers, listlessness) are signs to notify your doctor. In cases of severe diarrhea, doctors occasionally recommend supplements of an electrolyte solution, such as Pedialyte, in conjunction with nursing.

THE FIRST TWO MONTHS: WHAT'S NORMAL?

During the first two months you can expect your baby will nurse between 8 and 12 times a day, including at least once at night. If your baby sleeps four to six hours at a stretch at night or takes a three- to four-hour nap during the day, she will probably want to nurse often during the next few hours to make up for the meal she missed. The baby who is nursing less than eight times in a 24-hour period or who is sleeping longer than six hours at a stretch at night is typically the infant who fails to gain enough weight during the early weeks of nursing.

Generally, eight or more wet diapers a day are a sign the baby is getting enough milk. By two weeks, most nursing infants have regained their birth weight. A gain of at least an ounce a day is normal.

The breastfed baby typically has loose, watery, or seedy stools. During the first month most infants have at least one bowel movement daily. After the first month it is not uncommon for a baby to go several days without a bowel movement. As long as the baby seems comfortable there is probably no need for concern; your baby is unlikely to be constipated or underfed. The baby who is not getting enough to eat typically has small, and usually infrequent, brown or greenish stools and is gaining less than an ounce a day.

Many mothers continue to experience dripping or spraying milk during or between nursings. But some women stop leaking altogether after the first several weeks, and most gradually notice less leakage.

At some point during the first two months you will probably start to experience the sensations of milk let-down. You may notice this tingling, pins-and-needles feeling in your breasts just before or during a feeding or at any time your baby signals you with his cry.

Occasionally babies spit up after a feeding. Some babies spit up after every nursing. This is usually due to an immature digestive system; what comes up is normally just a few teaspoons. If your baby spits up more, the cause may be certain foods or beverages in your diet (see "Spitting Up and Vomiting," page 149, and "Fussiness, Colic, and Reflux," page 152). In any case, spitting up passes with time; until it does, keep a diaper or small towel handy.

A baby cries for any of a number of reasons. She may be hungry or tired, or she may just want to suck and be held. Sucking at the breast is soothing and comforting for her. Babies usually have a fussy period in the evening. Although many theories have been suggested to explain why this is, most babies are comforted by extra nursing. Try not to assume your milk is somehow lacking. Many mothers who interpret their babies' cries this way begin supplementing with formula and soon find the babies weaned. See "Fussiness, Colic, and Reflux," page 152, for more on why babies cry and how to cope with crying.

During the appetite spurts at about two to three weeks and six weeks of age, your baby may act more fussy than usual and want to nurse more often. After a few days of frequent nursing, your milk supply will increase to meet her needs and she will return to her usual nursing pattern.

Some babies cry hard, as if they were in pain, for prolonged periods every day. They are said to have *colic*, which is just a name for extreme irritability that continues day after day—for any of a number of reasons. Some cry at the breast or refuse nursing entirely. If your baby has colic symptoms, see "Fussiness, Colic, and Reflux," page 152.

You may have heard that tending to your baby each time she cries will spoil her or will reinforce her behavior and cause her to cry more often. Nothing could be further from the truth. Babies do not cry to exercise their lungs, but because they are in need of something. If your baby's needs are met in infancy she will develop a sense of security, and she will grow to trust in you and others as well.

During these early weeks, while you are learning about your baby, caring for his needs, and learning to breastfeed, you are apt to experience some feelings of concern, confusion, and perhaps even inadequacy regarding your mothering abilities. Motherhood and breastfeeding may not be exactly what you expected. Your baby's crying and the unpredictability of his sleeping and wakeful periods may be upsetting. The baby's nursing schedule (or lack thereof) and his many needs may make it impossible to feel organized or productive. Perhaps you are disappointed by the lack of help from your health-care providers. Early motherhood may also bring feelings of loneliness and isolation.

It is normal to have mixed feelings about nursing. Try to keep in mind that new motherhood brings a period of uncertainty and adjustment and that nursing, and mothering, gets easier with time.

SURVIVAL GUIDE

THE FIRST TWO MONTHS

CONCERNS ABOUT YOURSELF

Sore Nipples
Breast Pain
Plugged Ducts
Breast Infection (Mastitis)
Breast Abscess
Breast Lumps
Leaking Milk
Overabundant Milk
Lopsided Breasts
Nausea or Headache
Depression and Anxiety

CONCERNS ABOUT THE BABY

Spitting Up and Vomiting
Pulling Away from the
 Breast
Refusal to Nurse
Fussiness, Colic, and Reflux
Underfeeding

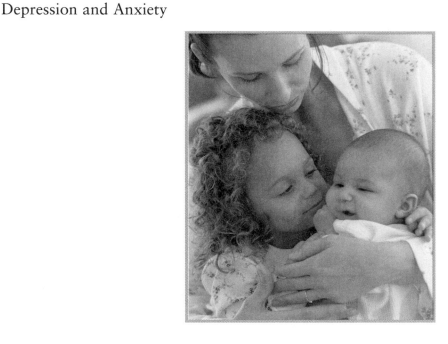

CONCERNS ABOUT YOURSELF

Sore nipples

It can certainly be discouraging when sore nipples persist beyond the first week. If this happens to you, review the information on sore nipples (page 50) in "Survival Guide: The First Week." It may be helpful to have your partner, friend, or lactation professional observe your latch-on technique and compare it with the descriptions of latch-on in "Positioning at the Breast," page 30. Don't discount the possibility that your nipples are irritated due to thrush or another dermatologic condition, as these are frequent causes of sore nipples.

If you have suddenly developed sore nipples after a period of comfortable nursing, the most likely cause is thrush. See "Thrush Nipples," page 53.

Painful, blanched nipples. Some women notice that their nipples become painful and blanched at the end of nursing sessions. Often this pain and blanching results from poor positioning of the baby at the breast. The compression of the nipples probably causes a vasospasm—a spasm in the blood vessels—preventing blood from getting to the nipples. You may be able to solve this problem by correcting your latch-on technique (review "Positioning at the Breast," page 30) and by applying warm compresses to the nipples right after nursing.

Sometimes vasospasm in the nipples results from Raynaud's phenomenon (formerly called Raynaud's syndrome), in which blood-vessel spasms, brought on by a drop in temperature, prevent blood from getting to a particular area of the body. Most commonly, Raynaud's phenomenon occurs in the fingers, typically when a person goes outdoors from a warm building on a cool day. In this case, the fingers turn white and the tips hurt. Raynaud's phenomenon affects as many as 22 percent of 21- to 50-year-old women and may be associated with illnesses such as rheumatoid arthritis.

When Raynaud's affects the nipples, it causes nipple blanching just after a feeding, probably because the ambient air is cooler than the inside of the baby's mouth. When the baby comes off the breast, the nipple is its usual color, but it very quickly turns white. This blanching is accompanied by burning pain. Then the nipple turns blue; this is caused by deoxygenation of the blood. As the blood starts flowing back to the nipple, the nipple returns to its normal color, and the mother may experience a throbbing pain. The nipple colors and types of pain may alternate for several minutes to an hour or more. The three-phase color change—from white to red to blue—suggests a diagnosis of Raynaud's phenomenon rather than poor positioning.

If you have Raynaud's phenomenon, avoiding cold is important. Your entire body needs to be kept warm. Breastfeed in a warm place, wear warm clothing, and avoid exposure to cold at all times. If you experience a painful vasospasm, applying warm, moist cloths to your nipples may help. Avoid smoking and caffeine.

Dietary supplements may help alleviate vasospasms caused by Raynaud's phenomenon. Some women have used a combination of calcium (2,000 milligrams per day) and magnesium (1,000 milligrams per day). So far, however, no studies have tested the effectiveness of this remedy. Jack Newman, a pediatrician, reports that vitamin B$_6$ often helps with Raynaud's phenomenon and is safe to use. He suggests a dosage of 150 to 200 milligrams once a day for four days. If the symptoms don't lessen in this much time, vitamin B$_6$ probably won't help at all, Newman says. But if the pain resolves, he suggests taking a reduced dose of 25 milligrams once a day until you are pain-free for a few weeks. If the pain returns with the smaller dose, you can return to the higher dose.

Various drugs have been investigated for the treatment of Raynaud's phenomenon. The most effective among them is nifedipine, which is primarily used to treat hypertension. Nifedipine is probably safe to use, since very little of the drug (less than 5 percent of the total dose) appears in the breast milk, and side effects in the mother are uncommon (the most frequent side effect is a headache). The usual dosage of nifedipine is one 30-milligram slow-release tablet per day for two weeks. If the nipple pain returns, as it does in about 10 percent of mothers, a second course can be taken. Women rarely require more than two or three courses.

Breast pain

For a variety of reasons, your breasts may begin to hurt during nursing or become perpetually tender or sore. If this happens, it is important to identify the cause so that any necessary action can be taken.

Engorgement can occur any time the breasts become overly full—when the baby misses a feeding, for example, or when he begins to sleep longer at night.

Most mothers begin noticing normal let-down sensations during these early weeks. Let-down may be experienced as a mild ache at the start of nursing or a tingling, pins-and-needles sensation.

A deep pain, often described as "shooting," that occurs just after nursing is thought to be related to the sudden refilling of the breast. These pains disappear after the first few weeks of nursing. Blocked nipple pores can also cause stabbing pains.

Pain during nursing, often described as burning or stinging, is usually associated with thrush. The nipples may be pinker than usual. Sometimes a rash may be visible. See "Thrush Nipples," page 53, for additional information on causes and treatment.

Plugged ducts
If you can feel a tender area or painful lump in your breast, the cause is probably a plugged milk duct. A plugged duct may be small or it may involve a large area of the breast that feels overly full and does not soften with nursing. The skin over the area may be reddened.

Occasionally a plug in one of the nipple openings blocks the milk flow and causes a backup of milk in the breast. If the nipple looks normal in color but you can see a white pimple ("bleb") on the face of the nipple, particularly right after the baby comes off the breast, the problem may be a plugged nipple pore. Plugged nipple pores are often associated with stabbing breast pain, especially right after nursing.

Plugged ducts are most common during the early weeks of nursing, but they can occur at any time during breastfeeding. They occur for a variety of reasons. During the early weeks and months of nursing, they frequently seem due to incomplete drainage of the breast. Mothers with high milk production, including those nursing twins, tend to be more prone to plugged ducts. Interrupting the baby's nursing to switch to the other breast before the baby signals that he is finished may lead to a plugged duct. A plugged duct may follow a missed feeding or a long stretch at night without nursing. Overly tight bras, especially underwire types, may obstruct milk flow and lead to plugged ducts. Baby carriers with tight straps can also cause this to happen.

For unknown reasons, plugged ducts seem to be more common during the winter months. Some breastfeeding specialists feel that mothers who drink an insufficient amount of fluids, who become slightly dehydrated due to a cold or flu, or who are overly fatigued may also be more susceptible to developing plugged milk ducts.

Any breast lump that does not get significantly smaller within a week should be examined by a doctor.

Treatment Measures for Plugged Ducts

1. Remove your bra if there is any question that it may be too tight or may be pressing into part of your breast.
2. Apply moist heat to the breast for 15 to 20 minutes before nursing.
3. Nurse frequently, at least every two hours. Begin each nursing on the affected breast.
4. Gently massage the breast just behind the sore area while nursing.
5. If you are following the preceding recommendations but notice no change in your breast after a feeding or two, try positioning the baby with his chin close to the plugged duct, if possible, to promote better drainage. If this doesn't work, get into the shower. With your breast well soaped, apply steady but gentle pressure behind the plugged area, pressing toward the nipple.
6. Increase your fluid intake so that you urinate more frequently.
7. When the blockage seems to be in the nipple, look for dried milk secretions or a clogged nipple pore, which may resemble a whitehead. If necessary, you can gently remove a visible plug from a nipple opening with a sterile needle. This may cause a little bleeding, but you probably won't feel any pain.
8. Be alert for signs of a developing breast infection—fever, chills, and achiness—so you can treat it promptly.

Breast infection (mastitis)

Up to 30 percent of all nursing women develop mastitis, or infection of the breast. It occurs most often in the first three months after birth, and, interestingly, it is more common during the winter months.

A breast infection is caused by bacteria, often the same ones normally present on the nipples and in the baby's mouth. A breast infection often follows an untreated cracked nipple or a plugged milk duct. It is more likely to occur when the baby (or a pump) is ineffective at draining the breasts. Other possible causes include poor-fitting bras, skipped feedings, infrequent changing of wet breast pads, anemia, stress, and fatigue.

Since mastitis causes flu-like symptoms, women sometimes mistake it for the flu. Headache, general achiness, and a reddened area of the breast are the early symptoms; they are usually followed with fever, typically over 101° F., chills, and weakness. Usually only one breast is affected; it becomes quite tender in the infected area.

Women who promptly apply moist heat to the breast and work on getting it as empty as possible may recover quickly without antibiotics, usually in two days. In one study of women with mastitis, half used no antibiotics, and none of them suffered complications (Riordan and Nichols, 1990). I have come to believe, however, that prompt treatment with antibiotics is indicated whenever a nursing mother has flu-like symptoms and a reddened breast, especially if she has a fever. Some women have permanently lost their milk production from the affected breast following a breast infection, usually when treatment has been delayed. Late treatment can also result in a breast abscess that may require surgical drainage. This risk is much greater if you are anemic.

Effective treatment with an antibiotic requires the right choice of antibiotic for the bacteria. The type of bacteria involved in mastitis is usually *staphylococcus aureus*, which is resistant to amoxicillin, penicillins G and V, and many other antibiotics. The two most effective classes of antibiotics against this organism are penicillins such as cloxacillin and dicloxacillin, which resist the enzyme that bacteria produce to inactivate other penicillins, and the cephalosporins, such as Keflex. Another frequently prescribed penicillin is Augmentin, an improved form of amoxicillin. Erythromycin, clarithromycin, azithromycin, and clindamycin are used in women allergic to penicillin. All of these antibiotics are safe to take while breastfeeding unless the baby is allergic to them (the allergy causes a rash).

With prompt and proper treatment the symptoms usually subside within 24 hours. It is most important to continue nursing frequently during this period; discontinuing nursing would slow healing and might lead to the development of a breast abscess. You don't need to worry that the baby will get ill, since the infection involves only the breast tissue, not the milk. Try to identify the probable cause of the infection so you can prevent a recurrence in the future.

Mastitis in both breasts, though rare, is sometimes a sign of B-streptococcal infection, which is transmitted by the infant to the breasts. When both breasts are affected, the baby's doctor should be promptly notified so that any necessary treatment of the infant can begin.

Treatment Measures for Mastitis

1. Go to bed, if you haven't already.
2. Remove your bra if you are more comfortable without it or if there is any question that it may be too tight or pressing into part of your breast.
3. Nurse frequently, at least every two hours, and begin each nursing on the affected breast. Giving up nursing could slow healing and lead to a breast abscess.
4. If nursing is too painful or if you suspect the baby isn't draining the affected breast well, begin pumping your breasts after or instead of nursing. Use a fully automatic pump and a double-pump kit, and pump approximately every two hours.
5. Call your doctor, who will probably prescribe antibiotics. Antibiotics should be taken for the entire time they are prescribed, even though the symptoms may disappear.
6. Increase your fluid intake so you notice an increase in urination.
7. Apply moist heat to the breast for 15 to 20 minutes before nursing and intermittently between feedings.
8. Monitor your temperature. Acetaminophen tablets (such as Tylenol) or ibuprofen (such as Advil or Motrin) may help reduce your fever and discomfort.
9. Consider taking vitamin C. Some women report that a dosage of 1,000 milligrams four times a day speeds healing and recovery.
10. After you have completed a course of antibiotics, watch for symptoms of yeast growth—thrush (see page 53) or diaper rash (see page 153).
11. See "Recurrent Plugged Ducts and Breast Infections" (page 204) if you have a recurrence.

Breast abscess

On very rare occasions, a breast infection may develop into an abscess. A breast abscess is an accumulation of pus walled off within the breast. It may occur when a mother stops nursing during a breast infection, when treatment for mastitis is delayed, or when a mother has trouble fighting off a breast infection because she is severely anemic.

A breast abscess should be suspected whenever mastitis symptoms are prolonged beyond a couple of days and a lump persists. The lump may be hard or soft but does not change with nursing. An abscess must usually be drained by a physician, either in an office or a hospital. After it is drained, recovery is rapid.

Some doctors are willing to avoid surgical drainage by performing a series of needle aspirations. This is much less invasive than opening the abscess to drain over a period of a couple of weeks.

The development and treatment of an abscess is usually a rather traumatic experience. You may be advised to stop nursing entirely, or you may doubt yourself whether you should continue. Although you need not abandon nursing completely, it may be suggested that you not nurse on the affected breast for the first few days after it is drained. In the meantime, you can use an electric pump to maintain your milk flow until the baby resumes nursing on both sides. The incision may leak milk for a short while, but it will heal and close over. I developed an abscess at six weeks after birth and went on to nurse successfully without any further difficulties.

Breast lumps

Lumps in the breast are very common during the early weeks and are usually related to lactation.

The breast may feel generally lumpy when it is overly full or engorged. A sudden tender lump is usually a sign of a plugged milk duct or, when accompanied with fever and flu-like symptoms, a breast infection. A lump that appears just before nursing and seems to get smaller or disappear afterward is probably a small cyst that fills with milk.

Whenever a lump shows no change in size for longer than a week, it should be examined by a doctor. It is probably a harmless cyst or benign tumor; cancer is rarely the cause. But breastfeeding women with persistent lumps have been found to have breast cancer, so see your doctor for a thorough breast exam as soon as possible. If further diagnosis is recommended, you don't need to wean your baby, although a doctor unfamiliar with the lactating breast may recommend weaning. Many women have undergone mammography, ultrasound, breast biopsy, and lump removal without any interruption of nursing. Feel free to get a second opinion whenever drastic measures are recommended.

Leaking milk

See "Survival Guide: The First Week," page 57, for basic information on leaking, dripping, and spraying milk.

After a few weeks of nursing you may notice that leaking diminishes or stops entirely. This need not be a cause for concern so long as the baby is continuing to nurse frequently and is gaining weight.

If continuing leakage is becoming bothersome, you might want to try stopping it by pressing your wrist or the heel of your hand against your nipples whenever they start to drip. You might also try LilyPadz, tacky silicone pads that can be worn without a bra (see Appendix A, page 244).

If leaking at night continues to be troublesome, you might try nursing the baby just before you go to sleep.

Overabundant milk

Some mothers seem to produce too much milk. Besides feeling weary of the jokes about being able to nurse twins, you may feel uncomfortably engorged much of the time. Leaking and spraying may be bothersome. Your baby may gasp and choke as the milk lets down.

Most women find this less of a problem after the first two months of breastfeeding. In the meantime, nursing your baby on just one side at each feeding should make your breasts feel more comfortable. When your baby is draining your breasts more completely they will feel less engorged, even though each is nursed on less often. Decreasing your fluid intake is not recommended. Nor is wearing plastic breast shells or pumping after or between feedings, either of which would probably increase, not decrease, milk production.

If your baby has difficulty nursing because the milk lets down forcefully, see "Pulling Away from the Breast," page 150. Refer to "Overabundant Milk," page 205, if you continue to produce milk in overabundance after two months.

Lopsided breasts

When one breast receives more stimulation than the other, milk production in that breast increases, commonly resulting in a lopsided appearance.

Providing more stimulation to the smaller breast will usually even out the size difference between the two. Start each feeding on the smaller side for a day or so. If your baby nurses there only a few minutes, encourage her to take the smaller breast again after she has nursed at the fuller one. As soon as your breasts become closer in size, you can begin alternating the breast at which the baby begins each feeding.

Nausea or headache

Rarely, a new mother experiences nausea when nursing her newborn. This is a biological phenomenon, not a psychological one; it is thought to be a gastric hormonal response to suckling. Eating something before nursing may help. Fortunately, nausea generally decreases in severity and frequency as nursing is established, and the problem usually disappears completely by six to eight weeks post partum.

Headaches in a new mother can have many causes: a drop in hormones in the first week post partum; low blood sugar; eye, dental, or sinus problems; allergies; or migraine. Several case reports in medical literature, however, have concerned "lactational headaches." These occur during feedings as the milk lets down and may be related to the hormone oxytocin. Some writers have said that pain relievers such as acetaminophen (Tylenol) and ibuprofen (Motrin, Advil) are helpful, and that these headaches gradually become less severe and stop by two months post partum. But other writers have described cases in which relief came only with weaning.

Another type of headache associated with lacatation occurs when one or both breasts are overfull. This type of headache may be a sign of an impending breast infection. Relief comes from draining the breasts well and heading off mastitis.

Regardless of the suspected cause of your headaches, you may want to consult with your doctor or a neurologist if they are frequent or severe. Keeping a headache log can be helpful in determining a diagnosis.

Depression and anxiety

Most women go through emotional changes after giving birth. Many new mothers experience moodiness, mild anxiety, or an occasional "blue" day during the first two weeks after delivery. These feelings are due to the sudden hormonal changes that follow birth, fatigue from labor and lost sleep, and stress that becoming a mother entails. But when emotional symptoms are severe, when they continue beyond the first two weeks after birth, or when they start later and last more than two weeks, they may indicate postpartum depression or anxiety. Many new mothers who complain that they are depressed or anxious are told that their feelings are normal and to be expected. This is not true. Postpartum emotional disorders are often misunderstood or unrecognized by family, friends, and health professionals.

As many as one out of every nine or ten new mothers experiences postpartum depression, postpartum anxiety, or both. Much rarer is postpartum psychosis, characterized by delusions, hallucinations, or extreme mental confusion. Postpartum emotional disorders are more common in women who have had a stressful pregnancy or difficult birth, previous psychological problems, or relationship difficulties. Occasionally, a thyroid disorder may mimic postpartum depression.

Symptoms of postpartum depression or anxiety usually include several of the following:

- Change in eating habits (poor appetite or overeating);
- Change in sleep pattern (difficulty falling or staying asleep, over-sleeping);
- Tenseness, nervousness;
- Panic attacks with physical symptoms such as shakiness, palpitations, shortness of breath, or lightheadedness;
- Fatigue or lack of energy;
- Poor concentration, forgetfulness, or confusion;
- Crying every day;
- Feelings of hopelessness;
- Withdrawal, lack of interest in usual activities;
- Excessive worry or guilt feelings;
- Recurrent disturbing thoughts or compulsive behaviors that cause distress or take up a great deal of time; and
- Failure to keep appointments.

Symptoms that call for immediate assistance from a mental-health professional include—

- Thoughts of suicide,
- Fears of harming the baby,
- Sounds and voices heard when no one is around,
- Thoughts that seem not your own or out of your control,
- Sleeplessness lasting 48 hours or longer,
- Inability to eat, and
- Inability to care for the baby.

For any woman suffering from postpartum depression or anxiety, I strongly recommend the book *This Isn't What I Expected: Recognizing and Recovering from Depression and Anxiety after Childbirth*, by Karen Kleiman and Valerie Raskin (see "Suggested Supplemental Reading"). Many women with mild cases have helped themselves without professional assistance. Try the coping measures that follow.

Coping Measures for Depression and Anxiety

1. Tell your partner, a supportive friend, or a relative how you are feeling. Although some people may not understand, you may find valuable support close by.

2. Talk to your doctor or midwife about how you are feeling. Ask about having blood tests done to make sure something else, such as a thyroid disorder, isn't the problem.

3. Call Depression After Delivery (800-944-4PPD) to find out whether there is a postpartum support group in your area.

4. Make getting extra rest a priority; being tired makes depression and anxiety worse. Nap when your baby naps. Maximize your baby's sleep stretches at night by feeding him every two to two and a half hours during the day and evening.

5. Enlist the help of others to relieve you of some mothering and household duties. Eliminate or lessen your daily chores until you are feeling better. If you want to do some chores, set minimal goals for yourself.

6. Maintain a well-balanced diet. If you have little appetite, fix small, nutritious snacks for yourself throughout the day. Avoid all caffeine and sugary foods and beverages; these are associated with worsening symptoms. Increase your intake of foods made up of complex carbohydrates, such as whole-grain breads and cereals, potatoes, rice, and pasta. Eat more fruits and vegetables. Using powdered milk or yogurt, wheat germ, and fruit or juice concentrate, you can make nutritious blender drinks. If you find it difficult to prepare food for yourself throughout the day, your pharmacist can recommend a high-calorie nutritional supplement such as Ensure or Sustacal.

7. Take time with your appearance every day. When you get up, make a point of getting dressed, fixing your hair, and putting on a little makeup, if you like it. Pamper yourself with a facial, a new hair style, or something new to wear. Looking good helps you feel better about yourself.

8. Get some exercise every day. Many people find that exercise has an antidepressant effect. Join an exercise or dance class; many offer free child care. Take a brisk walk every day with or without the baby.

9. Nurture yourself as much as possible. Take long bubble baths, get a massage, ask your partner to hold you, spend the afternoon watching a video or reading a light novel.

10. Make an effort to spend time with other adults. Invite friends over, join a postpartum group, or make friends with other mothers from your childbirth class. Your childbirth instructor may have additional suggestions. If you have just moved to the area, ask your pediatrician's or family practitioner's nurse for other resources.

If your distress is severe or unrelieved by these measures, consider seeking professional help. Low-cost mental-health care is available in most communities. If cost isn't an issue, ask your doctor, midwife, or childbirth educator to refer you to a therapist, ideally one who has a special interest in postpartum illness.

Depending on your symptoms, a therapist may recommend medication. Some antidepressants are safe to use during nursing; others may not be. One safe antidepressant is sertraline, which is sold under the trade name Zoloft; when nursing mothers take this drug, it is undetectable in their babies' blood. You may be tempted to try St. John's wort, now a popular remedy for depression. This herb, however, has not yet been proven safe to use during breastfeeding.

Unfortunately, many doctors who recommend that women wean their babies before taking antidepressants do so because they don't know about recent studies on the safety of particular drugs during breastfeeding. In Appendix C you'll find what information is available about the safety of various antidepressants. You may need to share this information with your doctor before coming to an agreement about what is best for you and your baby.

CONCERNS ABOUT THE BABY

Spitting up and vomiting

Spitting up small amounts of breast milk is common; some babies do this after almost every nursing. Recently, it has become common for doctors to diagnose these babies with "reflux" (see "Fussiness, Colic, and Reflux," page 152). Occasionally a baby may vomit what seems like an entire feeding. Although there may be no apparent cause, this can sometimes be traced to something the mother recently ate. Vomiting can also be a sign of infection. You will want to notify your doctor if the baby has a fever or if the vomiting continues.

When a baby continues vomiting forcefully after most feedings, you should suspect that either he is sensitive to something in your diet or he has pyloric stenosis. *Pyloric stenosis* is an obstruction of the stomach that typically develops at about two to four weeks of age.

Although this condition is most common in first-born males, it can occur in females. Typically the vomiting becomes progressively worse; the baby eventually stops gaining weight, or loses weight, and may become dehydrated. In the breastfed infant the condition may go undiagnosed longer than in the bottle-fed infant, since breast milk is digested much more easily than formula. The baby's weight may not be affected until the obstruction becomes nearly complete. Frequently waves can be seen moving across the baby's lower abdomen from the left side to the right just after a feeding and prior to vomiting. X-rays confirm the diagnosis. The obstruction is corrected with a relatively simple surgical procedure.

Breastfeeding can resume within a few hours after the obstruction is removed. At this time breast milk is especially good for the baby because of its digestibility. Some mothers notice a temporary reduction in the milk supply after the baby's surgery. Rest, frequent nursing, and switching the baby from side to side during the feeding usually reverse this situation.

Pulling away from the breast

Babies pull off the breast while nursing for a variety of reasons. Often it is because they have had enough to eat or they need to be burped. If your baby has a cold, she may pull away because she is having trouble breathing through her nose. Try to position her so her head is elevated more during nursing. A cool-mist vaporizer may help to thin the nasal secretions so she will breathe easier.

Some babies pull away from the breast gasping and choking as the milk suddenly lets down. This is usually a temporary problem; the baby gradually learns to keep up with the rapid flow of milk. In the meantime, positioning the baby differently may help. Try sitting the baby up, using the football hold, or lying on your back with the baby's head over you. Some mothers manually express or pump milk until the initial spray has subsided. If your baby pulls away from the breast and cries or refuses to nurse, see "Refusal to Nurse," as follows.

Refusal to nurse

If your baby pulls away from the breast crying or refuses to nurse, don't assume he is ready to wean. There are a number of possible reasons for such behavior, but when it persists it can frequently be traced to certain foods in the mother's diet to which the baby is sensitive. Typically this behavior starts when the baby is about two weeks old. He may also act fussy and have very frequent, sometimes greenish stools.

Other symptoms may include gassiness, redness around the rectum, a mild rash anywhere on the body, or a stuffy nose. Fussiness while nursing and refusal to nurse may occur sporadically or may increase as the day goes on. Although the baby refuses the breast, he may eagerly take breast milk from a bottle. The reasons for this are unclear.

In the past, these symptoms were generally referred to as colic. Parents were typically told simply to endure colic, since the causes were poorly understood and the syptoms were often ougrown by three to four months of age. Recently, however, the syndrome of fussiness and spitting up has been identified as gastroesophageal reflux, which is also known as GER or simply reflux. Babies with reflux cry after and in between feedings, fuss at the breast, and sometimes refuse to nurse. These reactions are most likely due to a painful irritation of the esophagus. (See "Fussiness, Colic, and Reflux," page 152.)

A baby who has developed a yeast infection (thrush) may also become fussy at the breast and refuse to nurse. Besides having a characteristic white coating on the insides of his lips, cheeks, or both, the baby with thrush may be gassy. There may also be a bright red, dotted or peeling rash around the baby's genitals or on your nipples. Your nipples may burn or itch.

Babies with ear infections also sometimes fuss at the breast and refuse to nurse. Although ear infections are less common in breastfed than in formula-fed babies, especially in the first two months after birth, even in this period an ear infection may accompany or follow a runny nose.

Occasionally a baby will refuse to nurse because his mother is wearing perfume or a scented deodorant.

When a baby has been fed supplemental formula and the milk supply has lessened, he may lose interest in the breast, preferring the immediate flow from the bottle.

Treatment Measures When the Baby Refuses to Nurse

1. As long as your baby refuses to nurse, express your milk every two to three hours so your supply will not be affected. Feed the baby by bottle.
2. See the next section, "Fussiness, Colic, and Reflux."
3. Check your baby's mouth and your nipples for signs of thrush. See "Thrush Nipples," page 53.
4. If you can find no reason for your baby's irritability and refusal to nurse, have a doctor examine the baby.

Fussiness, colic, and reflux

You may be surprised to learn how much crying a baby can do and how uncomfortable it can make you feel. The sound of a baby's cry is intended to be distressing, so adults will be alerted to his needs and answer them.

Many mothers tend to blame themselves for their babies' crying, wondering if their inexperience, nervous feelings, or milk supply is somehow responsible. Keep in mind that most babies fuss and seek out the comfort of the breast when they are tired, bored, lonely, or uncomfortable as well as when they are hungry. When babies are having appetite spurts, they increase their nursing frequency for a few days to stimulate increased milk production. If you are worried that the baby is not getting enough milk, have him weighed. A weight gain of an ounce a day or more means your baby is getting enough milk (see "Underfeeding," page 162).

Some babies are extremely irritable during the early weeks, with periods of intense crying. If your baby's crying makes you feel that something is wrong, trust your instincts. By all means have your baby examined by your doctor.

Outlined below are common reasons that babies cry, and suggestions for relieving their distress.

Fussiness. All babies have fussy periods during their early weeks. You will probably notice that your baby is more fussy at around two to three weeks and again at around six weeks, when most babies experience appetite spurts. Fussiness in the late afternoon or evening is typical.

Harvey Karp, a California pediatrician theorizes that much of the fussing babies do in the early weeks results from missing the uterine environment. In *The Happiest Baby on the Block: The New Way to Calm Crying and Help Your Baby Sleep Longer*, Dr. Karp suggests that parents calm their babies through the five Ss:

Swaddling. Many societies have used this technique to imitate the secure feeling of the womb during late pregnancy. A baby is wrapped tightly in a thin blanket with his arms down at his sides. Keeping the arms and hands secured keeps the baby from flailing them and makes him more receptive to the other four calming techniques.

To swaddle your baby, lay the blanket out flat, turn in a corner, and place the baby's neck on the folded edge. With the baby's right arm straightened at his side, pull the right corner of the blanket tightly over his body, and tuck it under his lower back on the left side.

With his left arm straight at his side, pull the bottom corner of the blanket up over the right arm and shoulder and tuck the blanket under his right side; don't worry about scrunching the baby's legs. Now wrap the left side of the blanket snuggly across his body.

Side or stomach position. Although it is now known that laying a baby to sleep on his stomach raises his risk of succumbing to Sudden Infant Death Syndrome, laying a baby on his back tends to make him startle—to extend his arms and cry out as if he feels he is falling backward. To prevent startling—or the Moro reflex, as it is sometimes called—swaddle the baby and lay him down to sleep on his side, or let him rest on his stomach over your lap or shoulder.

Sushing. Loud white noise calms a baby because it sounds like the flow of blood from the placenta. The louder a baby cries, the louder the sushing he needs. Hair dryers and vacuum cleaners work as well as vocal sushing sounds.

Swinging. Swinging in rapid, small movements is also reminiscent of uterine life. The swinging should be about two to three times a second. You can swing your baby by wearing him as you walk, by rocking him, or by using a baby swing (see "Coping Measures for Fussiness, Colic, and Reflux," page 162).

Sucking. Sucking is the final technique to use in relaxing a fussy baby. You can calm a baby who is upset but not hungry either by nursing or offering a pacifier. If your baby seems to need a great deal of comfort sucking, a pacifier may be appropriate. You can introduce one when your baby is between two and six weeks old. Before two weeks a pacifier could interfere with the establishment of breastfeeding, and after six weeks your baby might be much less willing to accept it.

Diaper rash. A baby may fuss a lot if she has a diaper rash. For an entire day, apply a zinc oxide ointment (such as Desitin); expose the baby's bottom to the air as much as possible, and leave off disposable diapers or plastic pants. The rash should improve dramatically, unless it is caused by yeast. A yeast diaper rash is a dotty, red rash or a peeling rash that resembles a mild burn, typically in the genital area.

Yeast infection. Although they are common in infants, yeast infections are frequently overlooked as the cause of excessive fussiness. A baby with a yeast infection usually shows signs in his mouth—on his inner lips or cheeks, and sometimes also on the tongue. This is known as thrush. The baby is typically very gassy, as the yeast is frequently present in the intestinal tract as well. The yeast may also cause a diaper rash, as described on page 153. The mother's nipples are often reddened; they may show a rash, and they may itch or burn. One nipple may be more affected than the other.

Nystatin suspension (Mycostatin) is probably the drug of choice if your baby has a yeast infection. Because the nystatin is swallowed, the yeast in the bowel will be eliminated. Treatment with gentian violet kills only yeast in the mouth and therefore is not recommended for the baby who is fussy and gassy unless the nystatin seems ineffective after several days of treatment. See "Thrush Nipples," page 53, for a complete discussion of treatment measures.

Nystatin ointment can be used to treat the baby's diaper rash; it can also be used on your nipples. If your baby has no rash it would not be unusual for one to appear shortly after treatment with the oral medication. If the baby does have a rash, don't be surprised if it gets worse during the first few days of treatment.

If the baby's stools are green, he may also be reacting to certain foods in his mother's diet. See "Colic and Reflux," below.

The baby's temperament. Every baby is born with her own distinct personality. Some babies tend to be quiet, whereas others are more active. Some babies are highly sensitive to their surroundings, overreacting to any sudden stimulation. They are tense and jumpy, and often fussy. They may go almost instantly from sleep to calm to full-blown crying. Once crying, they may be difficult to soothe. Although some of these babies need to be carried around or entertained continually, others may actually resist being held or cuddled.

Learning how to mother a highly sensitive baby takes time and patience. You will soon develop a sense of what your baby enjoys and what she does not, how much stimulation she can tolerate and how to help her settle down. If your baby does not enjoy touching, try not to take it personally. With time and a gradual increase in physical closeness, she will eventually be able to tolerate and enjoy being held. Most babies outgrow their early fussy months and grow to be happy children.

Colic and reflux. Colic is a catch-all term for unidentified infant discomfort characterized by periods of intense crying and apparent abdominal pain. Although the causes of colic have been much debated over the years, doctors have often dismissed it as something parents must simply endure until the baby is three to four months old, when the symptoms are expected to lessen or disappear. In the meantime, the baby is unhappy, and her mother may wonder if breastfeeding is to blame.

Recently, many babies who might in the past have been labeled colicky have been diagnosed instead with gastroesophageal reflux, which is also called simply reflux. Reflux is the backward movement of food and acid from the stomach into the esophagus and sometimes into the mouth and out onto your shirt. Nearly all babies have episodes of reflux; most parents consider it normal for their babies to "burp up" after feedings. Some babies who regurgitate frequently show no apparent discomfort. Others, however, seem to suffer painful heartburn, even if they don't spit up their milk.

The main reason babies spit up is that the lower esophageal sphincter isn't fully developed in infants. Also, babies take in a lot of milk relative to the size of their stomachs, and many also swallow a lot of air when they nurse or suck on a pacifier. When the baby burps, milk may come up with the air.

Breastfed babies generally have fewer and less severe episodes of reflux than bottle-fed babies. Sucking at the breast triggers peristaltic waves along the gastrointestinal tract; these muscular contractions help to move the milk down into the stomach and on to the small intestine. Also, human milk digests more completely and almost twice as fast as formula. The less time the milk spends in the stomach, the less opportunity there is for it to acidify before backing up into the esophagus. In addition, breastfed babies are generally fed in a more upright position than bottle-fed babies. Gravity may help to keep the milk and gastric acid in the stomach where they belong.

Still, breastfed babies can suffer painful reflux. Symptoms of this problem can include sudden or inconsolable crying, arching during feedings, refusing the breast or bottle, frequent burping or hiccoughing, bad breath, gagging or choking, frequent throat inflammation, poor sleep patterns, slow weight gain, frequent ear infections, and, less commonly, respiratory problems—wheezing, labored breathing, asthma, bronchitis, pneumonia, and apnea.

Some babies with reflux want to eat all the time and therefore may grow very fast, although it may seem as if they spit up all the milk they take in. On the way down breast milk is very soothing, as is sucking itself. But if a baby overfills her stomach, her reflux symptoms can worsen. For such a baby, it may be helpful to nurse on one breast at a time; the slower flow of milk may soothe the baby's heartburn without overfilling her stomach. Some mothers have reported that pacifiers help such babies.

Other babies with reflux seem to find nursing painful. They not only cry after and in between feedings, but they fuss at the breast and sometimes refuse nursings altogether. Oddly enough, they may take the same milk from a bottle that they wouldn't take from the breast.

Many parents try to minimize reflux by keeping their babies upright or semi-upright for 30 to 45 minutes after feedings. Recent research has found, however, that putting a baby in an infant seat (elevated to 60 degrees) actually increases reflux. Reflux is reduced, the studies have found, when the baby is laid on her left side or on her stomach. But putting babies to sleep on their stomachs has been associated with a higher rate of Sudden Infant Death Syndrome. Perhaps the best idea is to carry the baby on her left side in a sling, both to minimize reflux and to soothe the baby with the motion of your body. You might also try laying the baby stomach-down on your forearm; parents say that the pressure on the belly seems to be soothing.

Jostling or other rough or fast movement of a baby after feeding may add to the problem of reflux. Burp the baby before switching breasts, but don't jiggle her. Just hold her over your shoulder or sit her upright, and pat her back gently. Let her suck at the second breast until she falls asleep.

Some babies seem to suffer more with lower belly discomfort than with regurgitation and heartburn. Besides crying, these babies' symptoms may include gassiness; stools that are very frequent or green, mucous, or even bloody; and redness around the rectum. A baby may have a stuffy nose or a rash on her face or upper body. She may want to nurse all the time.

Although streaks of blood in a baby's stool or diaper rarely indicate an emergency, for a parent they are alarming, and when they appear it's a good idea to call to the baby's doctor. In most cases, however, blood in the stool results from either an anal fissure or a food intolerance. An anal fissure—that is, a small tear in the anus—usually results from constipation and straining during a bowel movement. Since exclusively breastfed babies cannot be constipated, anal fissures are unusual for them. A sensitivity or allergy to something in your diet is the more likely cause. Some doctors may say that a baby with bloody stools should be temporarily weaned from the breast and fed hypoallergenic formula instead of breast milk, but this is usually unnecessary. In most cases, the bleeding stops after the mother removes the offending food from her diet and the baby's gut has time to heal.

Something in your diet. Whether or not your baby has bloody stools, if she exhibits colic or severe reflux symptoms every day or nearly every day you should try writing down everything you have eaten and drunk during the past three days. Make notes, too, of any particularly fussy periods the baby has had during the past three days. If you are producing a lot of milk, also have your baby weighed to see how fast she is gaining. A baby who is gaining much more than an ounce a day may be having symptoms of what I call hyperlactation syndrome, which is described on page 160.

Most foods that bother breastfeeding babies, as either intestinal irritants or allergens, fall into one of several major food categories. When a baby has been fussy at particular times, a suspect food can often be identified by looking back one to two meal periods. If eating chocolate, say, seems to cause your baby's symptoms, you can try giving up chocolate and see if she does better. But because more than one food may be making your baby fussy, you might be wise to avoid

Thursday	
8:30 A.M. Grapefruit juice Prenatal vitamin Granola with milk Toast with butter	**10:30 A.M.-12:00 noon** Fussy, spitting up
12:15 P.M. Roast beef and cheese sandwich, with mayonnaise and lettuce Potato chips Milk	**2:00 P.M.-5:00 P.M.** Crying
3:00 P.M. Pineapple juice	
6:45 P.M. Chicken-green pepper stir-fry Spinach and mushroom salad, Italian dressing Rice Milk	
8:15 P.M. Chocolate frozen yogurt	**11:30 P.M.-2:00 A.M.** Very fussy, vomited

Sample chart of a mother's diet and her baby's reactions.

all of the commonly offending foods for a while, then reintroduce them to your diet one by one. This way, you'll know exactly what bothers your baby.

Completely eliminating all of the following foods for three days may bring speedy relief to your fussy baby. Be sure to check the ingredients in any commercially processed food before eating or drinking it.

- *Chocolate and spices.* The major offender in chocolate is theobromide; even in small amounts, this ingredient is a potent irritant in the digestive tract of many infants. In the example given, the chocolate frozen yogurt was probably responsible for this baby's (and mother's) difficult night. Many spices and other strong flavorings, including cinnamon, chiles, garlic, and curry, can also bother young infants.

- *Citrus.* A frequently overlooked cause of digestive disturbances is citrus fruits and their juices. Oranges, lemons, limes, tangerines, and grapefruits can all bother a baby's intestines. Other strongly acidic fruits, such as pineapples, kiwis, and strawberries, affect many babies similarly. In the chart, the mother had grapefruit juice at breakfast and pineapple juice in the afternoon. Her baby may have been bothered by these.

- *Gas-producing vegetables.* Certain vegetables can also cause temporary digestive problems for young babies. These include onions, broccoli, cauliflower, brussels sprouts, cabbage, bell peppers, and cucumbers. Prepared mustard can cause a similar reaction. Onions, an ingredient in so many dishes, can cause gastric upset for a baby even when they are cooked, ingested in small amounts, or eaten as onion powder. The stir-fry dish in the chart contained one of these offending foods.

- *Cow's milk.* Some infants are allergic to cow's milk and cow's milk products, including cheese, yogurt, sour cream, cottage cheese, and ice cream. Researchers have estimated that nearly half of all cases of severe reflux and colic are associated with an allergy to cow's milk. If a baby is truly allergic to cow's milk products, cutting back on how much you have will probably not eliminate the baby's symptoms. You must eliminate from your diet all dairy products, including those in commercially processed foods like creamed soups, certain types of salad dressings, and puddings; cow's milk may be identified as "casein" or "whey" on the label. Many infant formulas are made from cow's milk. The baby in the chart may or may not be reacting to dairy products.

If possible, do without medications and dietary supplements while you're avoiding these four food categories. Laxatives taken by a nursing mother can disturb her baby's intestinal tract. Aspirin and the chemical phenylpropanolamine, a decongestant, can make a baby fussy; both of these drugs are in many headache and cold remedies. Certain dietary supplements taken by the mother or given directly to the baby, such as Vitamin C, brewer's yeast, and fluoride, have been known to cause colic symptoms. Fluoride is very helpful in preventing cavities, but is best delayed until the baby is six months old.

During the three days of eliminating all the commonly offending foods from your diet, write down what you eat and drink along with observations of your baby. If the baby has particularly difficult times, look back one to two meal periods, or about two to eight hours before the symptoms began, and try to identify any suspect foods. You may find that you ate something forbidden without realizing it, or perhaps another food seems to be at fault. Other foods that can cause reactions include tomatoes, eggs, peanuts and peanut butter, corn and corn syrup, wheat (in breads, crackers, cookies, cakes, and noodles), soy (the basis of some infant formulas and an ingredient in many processed foods), apples, and bananas. If you decide to eliminate any one of these foods, you should continue to avoid the original four food categories, too. More than one food group may be affecting your baby.

If your baby is much better after the three days, and having very few fussy periods or other symptoms, try adding milk products back into your diet. Have a lot of milk products early in the day and then watch the baby for 24 hours. If the baby reacts, avoid milk products completely for the next couple of days. After this period, you might experiment with small amounts of milk, cheese, yogurt, or ice cream to see which of these, if any, your baby can tolerate, and in what quantity. Although some babies cannot tolerate any milk products, others do fine when their mothers have hard cheese, and some can tolerate small amounts of any milk products as long as their mothers take them only once every few days. (If you must cut dairy products from your diet completely, be sure you are taking sufficient calcium in another form; see pages 122–123). Every few days thereafter, add another food category to your diet, eating a lot at a time. If the fussiness recurs, eliminate the offending food category from your diet again. Continue adding food categories until you have tested all the foods that you had eliminated. Again, more than one food may be a problem for a very sensitive baby.

Hyperlactation syndrome. Recently researchers have identified a kind of colic that is characterized by gassiness, frequent stools, spitting up, and general discomfort and fussiness (Woolridge and Fisher, 1988). Although these babies may seem to be allergic to something in their mother's diet, they show little or no improvement with the elimination of common allergens. Typically these babies nurse frequently from both breasts and are gaining more than an ounce per day. Their mothers often have overabundant milk supplies.

Some lactation professionals refer to these symptoms as Overactive Let-down Syndrome. In fact, the underlying cause of the colic is thought to be the baby's disproportionate intake of the low-fat foremilk, the milk that is available early in the feeding. When a baby consumes large amounts of foremilk and little of the fatty hind milk, his stomach rapidly empties, dumping excess lactose into the bowel. This results in increased fermentation and colic symptoms.

Relief of the colic is achieved by getting the baby to empty one breast at each feeding so that he receives not only the foremilk but the fatty hind milk too. The baby should be allowed to nurse from the first breast until he spontaneously pulls away satisfied. He should not be interrupted at any point to be switched over to the second breast. Some authorities feel that until the colic subsides the baby should be offered just one breast per feeding and should be limited to that side for one and a half to two hours before nursing on the other side.

When nothing else works. Whether your baby has painful reflux or other colic symptoms, the extreme stress of caring for her may make you consider another feeding method in hopes that the symptoms will lessen. Keep in mind that these conditions usually improve without any such change. Switching to formula, in fact, might well make the problem worse instead of better. Continuing to breastfeed will provide important health benefits for both you and your baby and, most important, a strong bond that can help you both get through this difficult time.

Some doctors recommend thickening milk with cereal for babies who suffer with reflux or colic, on the theory that heavier food stays down better. But there is no proof that this helps; in fact, adding cereal to a baby's milk may slow the emptying of her stomach, increase episodes of reflux, and possibly cause choking. Regurgitated solids are more irritating than regurgitated human milk, and if bits of cereal are aspirated into a baby's lungs they can cause pneumonia. Besides, cereal replaces rather than supplements breast milk in a baby's diet, and it can thus cause a decrease in the milk supply. Since many babies with severe reflux or colic have allergies, introducing cereal to them early can lead to fussing at the breast, refusal to nurse, and early weaning.

Medical tests for reflux and other digestive disorders are rarely advised unless the baby shows signs of poor growth, severe choking, or lung disease. The best test for severe reflux is the pH probe, in which a tube is put down the baby's throat to measure the acid level at the bottom of the esophagus. Less invasive is the barium swallow, in which the baby drinks a barium mixture, an X-ray is taken, and then the X-ray is examined for any blockage or narrowing of the stomach valves that may be causing or aggravating the condition. The X-ray, however, will not identify whether a baby's stomach contents are more acidic than normal or if the esophagus has been damaged by reflux. Damage to the esophagus is determined through a more invasive procedure, endoscopy with biopsy. All of these tests should be used cautiously; they do not always provide conclusive results, and they are stressful for both the baby and her parents.

Many doctors try medication, without doing any of these tests, to see if the medication will lessen the baby's symptoms. There are three kinds of medication for reflux. First are the calcium-based antacids, which neutralize stomach acid without known side effects. Among these, Mylanta Supreme is available over the counter (so are Mylicon drops, but they don't seem to help). These medications are given right after feedings.

Second are medications that suppress acid production in the stomach. These include cimetidine (Tagamet), famotidine (Pepcid), ranitidine (Zantac), and "acid blockers," which prevent all acid production. Among acid blockers, omeprazole (Prilosec) and lanseprazole (Prevacid) are approved for use in children. Since not all children react the same way to these drugs, you may have to try two or more before you find one that works well. It may take about two weeks before you can tell whether a particular drug works.

The third group of medications for reflux increase motility—that is, they improve the muscle tone of the digestive tract to keep the food moving through it. Metoclopramide (Reglan) is the motility drug currently used in the United States. It can cause gastric cramping and diarrhea. The long-term use of this drug in children (that is, over a period of weeks) hasn't been well studied; in fact, there are concerns about its long-term use in adults.

Needless to say, a baby with colic or severe reflux may sleep poorly and fuss a great deal. She may need to be held upright most of the time. She may deprive her mother of sleep and, by refusing the breast, make her feel rejected. The risks of postpartum depression and even child abuse are higher when a baby has severe reflux or colic. Since this can be a very challenging period even for the most stable family, it is important that you get emotional support, find practical help, and limit your commitments until the problem passes.

Coping Measures for Fussiness, Colic, and Reflux

1. Offer your breast—it is a source of comfort as well as nourishment for your baby.
2. Try a pacifier. Pacifiers are soothing to many babies who need a lot of extra sucking, who are fussy, or who have difficulty calming themselves. If your baby won't take a pacifier at first, try different kinds.
3. Be sure to burp your baby frequently while he nurses or sucks on a pacifier.
4. Try swaddling your baby tightly in a light blanket.
5. Soothe both yourself and the baby with a warm bath.
6. Most babies love motion. Try walking, using a baby pack, sling, or stroller. Rocking can also be comforting—borrow a rocking chair if you don't already have one. You can put a small baby in a baby swing if you bolster him with towels or blankets. Most babies are lulled to sleep by car rides.
7. White noise may calm a crying baby. Try helping him sleep by turning on a radio or a tape recording of a humming car or vacuum cleaner, or by placing an aquarium near the baby's bed.
8. Consider sleeping with the baby, if you aren't doing so already.
9. Take a short break from the baby each day. Your partner might play with him while you take a bath, go for a walk, or visit a friend.
10. Find another mother who has a fussy baby. There's nothing like a friend who really understands.

Underfeeding

For any number of reasons, you may wonder if your baby is getting enough to eat. It may be that he seems to be nursing all the time or is especially fussy. Most young infants want to nurse eight to twelve times in each 24-hour period. Nursing this often is normal and seldom reflects a poor milk supply. You can't tell whether your baby is getting enough breast milk by offering him a supplemental bottle of water or formula after nursing. Most babies will take one to two ounces if it is offered, even when they have had enough milk from the breasts. The baby is probably getting enough milk if—

- he is nursing at least eight times in a 24-hour period,
- he is nursing 10 to 45 minutes at each feeding and seems content after feedings,
- he has several periods of swallowing during each feeding,
- your breasts feel softer or lighter after the baby has nursed, and
- your baby is having bowel movements every day during the first month.

If any of these statements is false, have your baby weighed. Even if all are true, have your baby weighed if you need the reassurance. The nurse in your baby's doctor's office should be happy to do this for you.

Between the fifth day and the end of the third or fourth month after birth, a baby should gain an ounce every day. A weight gain of an ounce a day reflects an adequate milk intake. If your baby was weighed at any time after the fifth day, you can see whether he has gained enough by weighing him again now. If he hasn't been weighed since the fifth day, consider that by 10 to 14 days of age most babies have regained their birth weight. If your baby is two weeks old and weighs less than his birth weight, he probably needs more milk. If your baby is two weeks old and weighs more than his birth weight, he is probably getting plenty of milk. If you have any doubt about how much the baby is gaining, weigh him again in a couple of days.

Inadequate weight gain usually occurs when a baby has had trouble latching on or nursing vigorously during the period of initial engorgement in the first week, or when nursing has been infrequent. Underfeeding often occurs to the group of mothers and babies listed in "Babies Who May Not Get Enough," page 39. This problem can also occur when a newborn has a faulty suck, when a mother has used a nipple shield over her nipple for nursing, and, certainly, when a baby is sick. Some laxatives, when taken by the mother, can cause a baby to have excessive bowel movements and to lose weight or gain too slowly even if he is taking enough milk. A baby who gains weight slowly or not at all after gaining well at first may be suffering with painful reflux. Some babies with reflux limit their milk intake because of the discomfort of heartburn (see "Fussiness, Colic, and Reflux," page 152).

Usually a baby's failure to latch on or suck well during the early weeks quickly leads to low milk production. The solution is to build the milk supply by pumping after nursing, and to feed the baby the expressed milk along with any necessary formula.

Treatment Measures for Underfeeding

1. If possible, see a lactation professional.
2. To estimate the amount of milk you are producing and to increase your milk supply, rent a fully automatic electric breast pump (see Appendix A, page 243). Any other pump would be inadequate for accurately estimating milk production and would be less helpful in increasing your milk supply.
3. Estimate your milk production by pumping your breasts instead of nursing. If you are pumping one breast at a time, pump each twice, for a total pumping time of 20 to 25 minutes. If you have a double-pump kit, use it for a total of 12 to 15 minutes. Feed this milk and any necessary formula to your baby. (See Appendix B to determine how much milk your baby needs at each feeding.)

   Exactly two hours after completing the first pumping, pump again. This time you may get less milk than in the first pumping. Multiply the number of ounces collected at this *second* pumping by 12. This will give you an estimate of how much milk you are producing over a 24-hour period; if you collected $1\frac{1}{2}$ ounces, for example, you are producing about 18 ounces per day.

   Now you can compare the baby's daily milk requirement, as listed in Appendix B, with your milk production. For example, if you estimate that your baby needs 21.4 ounces per day and your milk production is 18 ounces per day, the baby needs about $3\frac{1}{2}$ ounces of formula per day until your milk production increases.

   If you determine that you have enough milk for your baby and yet he has not been gaining well, it may be that he is not taking all of the milk available at some or many of his feedings. This can happen with newborns who were born prematurely, who tend to drift off to sleep while nursing, who have sucking difficulties, or who suffer with painful reflux. In such a case, you'll still want to take the steps that follow, feeding your baby expressed breast milk (rather than formula) after nursing until his feeding skill improves.

4. After you have estimated your milk production, go back to nursing your baby at least eight times in every 24 hours. This may mean waking him for feedings. Nurse him every two and a half hours during the day and evening (counting from the start of one nursing to the start of the next) and every three to four hours in the night, for 10 to 15 minutes on each breast. (I suggest limiting the nursing to this amount of time so that the entire nursing-pumping-supplementing session can be completed in 40 to 50 minutes.) Frequent short nursings are more effective in increasing milk production than infrequent lengthy ones.

5. Pump your breasts right after each nursing to stimulate further milk production. If you're pumping one breast at a time, pump for five minutes on each side, and then pump each breast a second time for a few minutes. Pumping both breasts at once not only takes less time but increases milk production faster. Use a double-pump kit for 5 to 10 minutes after nursing.

6. Right after pumping, offer the baby whatever breast milk you've collected along with any necessary formula. If the baby needs supplemental formula, divide the total amount needed by the number of feedings the baby is getting each day (usually eight). For example, the baby needing 3$\frac{1}{2}$ ounces of formula could take about $\frac{1}{2}$ ounce after each of his eight daily nursings. The goal is to offer about the same amount of milk and formula at each feeding so that he wants to nurse at regular intervals.

   Many lactation consultants, fearing the bottle would interfere with the baby's ability at the breast, suggest that a baby be supplemented with a nursing supplementer, cup, eye dropper, or soft tube taped onto the feeder's finger. If one of these methods is recommended to you and it works well, then continue with it. But if you find it too frustrating or time-consuming, use a bottle. After the first few days of nursing, using a bottle for supplemental feedings rarely causes latch-on or sucking problems.

7. To stimulate even greater milk production, try fenugreek. Take fenugreek capsules, which are sold in health-food stores, two or three at a time, three times a day. See "Treatment Measures for Underfeeding," page 77.

8. Weigh your baby every few days to be sure that he is gaining well. After each weighing, re-estimate his milk needs, since as he gains weight his milk needs will increase. Re-estimate your milk production, too. Two hours after your last pumping, use the breast pump instead of nursing, and figure your milk production as explained in item 3. Hopefully your milk production will have increased enough that you can decrease or even eliminate any formula supplementation.

9. Consider taking a pharmaceutical drug—metoclopramide (Reglan) or domperidone (Motilium)—to stimulate milk production. See "Relactation," page 94.

10. Once your baby is gaining well, his nursing seems more vigorous, and he is receiving supplements only of your breast milk, try eliminating some of the supplement. For a few days, offer half of the milk that you are expressing to the baby, and freeze the rest. If the baby continues to gain well, keep pumping, but don't offer the baby any of the pumped milk. Once the baby is gaining an ounce a day without any supplement, you can gradually stop pumping. Continue to have your baby weighed weekly.

If treatment fails. It is frightening to realize that your baby is not getting enough to eat. Although the technique just described usually ensures a weight-gaining baby and higher milk production within several days, occasionally these measures won't work. Sometimes, when breast engorgement has been severe and little milk has been removed during the first week, the decline in milk production is difficult to reverse.

In unusual instances, a mother fails to produce milk. This sometimes happens to women who have had breast surgery, particularly when the surgical incision is around the areola (see "Nursing after Breast Surgery," page 86), or who have insufficient glandular (milk-producing) tissue, or "hypoplastic" breasts (see "Medical Reasons for Not Breastfeeding," page 85).

In any of these situations, lack of support from family, friends, and health professionals can only make matters worse. But even with all of the best information and support, things sometimes don't turn out as we hope. If you have given nursing your best, but finally end up having to bottle-feed, you have not failed as a mother. Be proud of your efforts to nurse, and concentrate on providing your baby with all of the cuddling and loving that you can. Detailed information about formula and bottle feeding can be found in *The Nursing Mother's Guide to Weaning* (see "Suggested Supplemental Reading").

Some mothers who can't produce enough milk have found that continuing to nurse with a nursing supplementer has been a rewarding, worthwhile experience. Others have found nursing supplementers to be cumbersome and frustrating. Another option, particularly if the baby has become frustrated at the breast, is to first bottle-feed and then nurse. "Comfort nursing"—nursing after or between bottle feedings, or during the night—may be a pleasant experience for both mother and baby.

5 TRAVELING TOGETHER, BEING APART

Today's nursing mother is out and about, taking care of business, enjoying the company of friends, returning to work or school, taking time out for fun. In many ways, nursing simplifies life considerably. With the increasing acceptance and popularity of breastfeeding, more and more mothers are able to nurse their babies while participating in a wide variety of activities.

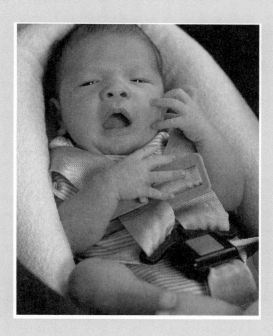

TAKING THE BABY ALONG

Your nursing baby can go with you almost anywhere—and with a lot less hassle than you would face if you were fussing with formula and bottles.

You may feel comfortable nursing in the presence of family or friends you are visiting, or you may be a bit uneasy. You can always retreat to the bedroom, of course, but that's not much fun. Learning to nurse discreetly and without embarrassment will put most people at ease. You might want to practice ahead of time getting the baby on your breast with a blanket or shawl draped over your shoulder and the baby's head. If you wear a shirt or a sweater you can pull up, or if you unbutton your blouse from the bottom, you will expose less of yourself. Most maternity shops carry a line of attractive tops and dresses designed for discreet nursing. Try nursing in front of your partner or in front of a mirror so you'll know what others will see.

If you are going out for the day or spending a few hours in town, you may want to nurse just before you leave. A couple of diapers and a few moist wipes in a sandwich bag, and you're off. If you are using a cloth baby carrier, you may find it easier to put it on before you go.

After a couple of hours out, look around for a comfortable place to sit with your baby. Many mothers feel comfortable nursing in public places and are hardly noticed when they do so. Some stores and restaurants have dressing rooms or pleasant restrooms where you may prefer to feed the baby.

Mothers appreciate the ease of taking long trips with their nursing babies. Most young infants travel well in a car. (Of course, the baby should always ride in a car seat approved for safety, no matter how short the trip.) You will want to stop every few hours for nursing and a diaper change. If the baby's car seat faces backward, you may be able to manage nursing while sitting in the back seat next to her.

The older baby may be less happy in the car seat for long periods. Whenever possible try to start long stretches in the car just before nap time. Try hanging some of the baby's toys on her car seat or keeping a bag of toys and other fun things in the back seat.

If you are planning to fly, you might try to reserve bulkhead seating; this will give you extra space. Try to choose a flight that is lightly booked. This way you are more likely to get an empty seat next to you for more room and privacy. Nursing during takeoff and landing will help the baby's ears adjust to the changing air pressure. If you must fly when the baby has a cold, give her a safe decongestant an hour before takeoff.

BEING APART

OCCASIONAL SEPARATIONS

Any number of situations may come up in which you must be separated from your baby—an evening out, perhaps, a family or career obligation, or a stay in the hospital.

When you plan to be away from the baby for just a few hours, you can manually express or pump some milk for him ahead of time. The best time to collect milk is just after nursing, especially if the baby has nursed from just one breast, or after your first morning nursing. In this way you will not lessen the amount of milk available for the baby at his next feeding. Getting an ounce or so after the baby nurses is typical. You will need to collect milk several times for each feeding you'll miss, as most young babies take about three to four ounces at a bottle feeding. If you will be away longer than four to five hours, bring the pump along; you will need it to prevent engorgement and to keep up milk production (see "Expressing Milk," page 175, and "Collecting and Storing Your Milk," page 186).

If you will be separated from the baby for a day or longer, you may be able to store enough milk for him ahead of time. If not, you can substitute a commercially prepared formula. While you are away, try to pump at least every two and a half to three hours. A rental electric pump may be more convenient than other kinds, and also is most effective for keeping up your milk supply. If possible, freeze the milk you pump while you are apart so that it can be used later.

Hospitalization of a nursing mother rarely necessitates weaning, even though some doctors advise it. Some hospitals have electric breast pumps available for nursing mothers. If your hospital doesn't, you can rent a pump and take it with you, or have one brought in. You may be able to arrange for the baby to be brought in for nursing visits, or even for the baby to stay with you (providing you, a family member, or a friend can care for him). Try to express your milk frequently to maintain your milk supply. Ask the nursing staff to refrigerate your milk so that it can be taken home for your baby.

Questions may arise about the safety of medications you need to take in the hospital. Although most medications pass through the breast milk, the majority are safe for nursing babies. Occasionally, a doctor may be unsure whether a given medication is safe for a baby and so recommends weaning when the question arises. You can check the safety of the drug yourself in Appendix C. If a drug is not considered safe for a nursing baby, you can continue to pump your milk, discarding it until the medication is no longer required.

RETURNING TO WORK OR SCHOOL

Not so long ago, a new mother planning to return to work might never have considered nursing her baby or would have decided to wean near the end of her maternity leave. Today, with the growing number of working women and the increasing awareness of the many benefits breastfeeding offers, more and more mothers are choosing to nurse their babies while continuing with their careers.

Your extra efforts to continue nursing are well worthwhile. The cost of formula aside, breastfed babies are generally healthier. The less your baby is sick, the less time you must spend away from work or school. Nursing also saves you time and energy, which is especially important when you are combining the responsibilities of employment and family. Perhaps most important, nursing helps you maintain the close, loving relationship you have with your baby. Many mothers who work outside the home or attend school feel that breastfeeding offers emotional compensation for the hours that must be spent apart. The security of your breast comforts the baby and helps make the time you are together special and rewarding for both of you.

WORK OPTIONS

Although there may be no question in your mind that you will be returning to work or school after your baby is born, you are lucky if you have some flexibility in determining the length of your maternity leave. Your time at home after giving birth is important for both you and the baby: it is the time in which you will get to know each other and form a special tie between you. It will also be a time for you to rest and recover from the physical stress of the birth process. Some women need a little while, and some need a long while, before they are ready to add the demands of work or school. Breastfeeding experts have noted that mothers who stay home for 16 weeks or longer experience fewer difficulties maintaining their milk supply once back at work.

Because you cannot know just how you will feel after you deliver, explore what options may be open to you ahead of time. Depending on your financial situation and your work demands, you may be able to arrange for an extended leave, beyond the usual six to eight weeks. Or you may be able to arrange to work at home, return to work part time, take fewer classes, or share your job with another person. Each of these options has worked well for many mothers.

Part-time work offers many advantages to the nursing mother. Fewer hours apart means fewer missed feedings, lower child care costs, and generally less hardship for both mother and baby.

Your employer also benefits by agreeing to shorter hours. Replacing an employee is time consuming and costly, especially if she has special skills that are an asset to the organization. Besides, part-time employees are known to be just as productive as those who work full time, if not more so. They tend to stay out sick less often, and they generally waste less time when they are at work. Part-timers can also help to reduce the overtime hours employers must pay for. You might agree to come in fewer hours each day, or have fewer full-hour days. Both arrangements have advantages and drawbacks for the nursing mother.

Of course, part-time work also means part-time pay. Perhaps the only choice for you is full-time work. Still, a somewhat flexible arrangement may be possible. With a "flextime" schedule, you might work eight hours a day but remain free to start earlier or later than normal. This system could allow you to spend a leisurely morning with the baby and perhaps get a few chores done. You might also be able to reduce the number of hours that the baby must be left with someone else if your partner can pick her up after work.

Some mothers arrange to take their babies to work with them. Although this is not possible for most women, it can be managed in some work settings. Another option is child care at the work site. Some employers and employees have found this to be an ideal arrangement. If you work with other parents of infants or small children, it might be well worth looking into this possibility.

Another possibility is having the baby brought to you for nursings, or going to the baby yourself during your lunch hour. Usually, the major obstacle in having the baby come to your work place is finding someone willing and able to bring her. If you choose to spend your lunch hour with the baby, you will need to find child care close to your work place. Combining your coffee breaks with your lunch hour may give you enough time to leisurely manage travel time, nursing, and eating.

CHOOSING A CAREGIVER

Finding just the right person to care for your baby can make all the difference in your state of mind while you are away. You may have the good fortune of relying on your partner or another loving relative to provide child care. Although this can be an ideal arrangement that makes the separation easier on both mother and baby, for most of us it is not an option.

If you will be shopping for a caregiver, be sure to start early so you can take your time. You may prefer that the caregiver come to your home, or that you take the baby to her. If you decide on the latter arrangement, try to locate a caregiver who lives close to your place of work or school. This will help you minimize the time you and your baby are apart and will be more convenient if you decide to nurse during your lunch breaks. You may prefer someone who will care for your baby alone, or you may be willing to share the caregiver's services with others.

Let each prospective caregiver know about your nursing relationship and your own particular style of caring for the baby. Be sure to ask for the names and telephone numbers of other families whose children she has cared for in the past or is caring for now. It's also a good idea to try to find out if she can make a long-term commitment to your baby; having to suddenly find a replacement can be upsetting for both you and your baby. If she cares for other children, try to schedule your meeting for when they will be present. This will give you the opportunity to observe firsthand the caregiver's style, and to see whether your baby would receive enough individual love and attention in the setting. In some states, child-care providers are licensed and limited in the number of infants and children they can care for. Feel free to ask about this.

In making your final choice of who will care for your baby, trust your intuition. If something doesn't feel quite right, look elsewhere. Before making a final commitment, be sure to discuss how you will handle illness (either your baby's or the caregiver's), who is to be called in an emergency, how much advance notice is necessary if the baby will be absent or late, fees and when they will be due, and any written agreements.

You may consider having the baby spend several hours or a full day with the caregiver a week or so before you go back to work or school. Such a "trial run" may be reassuring for you, or you may feel, as many mothers do, that the first separation should occur only when the situation demands it.

EXPRESSING MILK

If you will be missing one or more feedings while you are away at work or school, you should plan to express your milk. This will help to prevent engorgement and, more important, to maintain your milk supply. The milk you express can be used later to feed your baby while you are away. If you leave your baby for longer than four to five hours three or more times a week and do not express your milk, particularly if your baby is less than eight months old, your milk supply will probably diminish.

How often you should express milk depends on the age of your baby, how long you will be apart, and how often the baby nurses while you are together. Young babies normally nurse at least seven times in 24 hours; emptying the breast this often is necessary to maintain adequate milk production. If your baby is less than four months old, then, plan on expressing milk every two and a half to three hours while away.

Four- to seven-month-old babies typically nurse at least seven times a day. If your baby is this age, express milk often enough so that, with pumping and nursings, your breasts are emptied seven times in each 24 hours. If your five-month-old nurses frequently during the day and twice at night, you may not need to express milk while you work four hours a day, unless you prefer that your baby receive only breast milk when you are apart.

A baby who is eight months old or older may be nursing often or just a few times a day. Whether or not to express milk at this age depends not only on how much time you spend away from your baby, but also on whether he is eating a wide variety of solid foods and how you feel about providing formula instead of breast milk.

If you decide against expressing milk, your baby will need a commercially prepared formula for missed nursings during the first year.

Manual expression

Many mothers feel that expressing milk by hand is more convenient and natural than using a pump. You can learn this technique while nursing, practicing on the free side when the baby stimulates the milk to let down. Place a towel in front of you to catch the spray as you get started. Position your thumb and index finger about one

▲ *When using hand expression, catch the milk in a cup or any other clean container.*

and a half inches behind the nipple, where the milk sinuses are located. Push your fingers straight back toward your chest and then squeeze them together with a slight rolling motion, lifting the nipple outward. Avoid sliding your fingers away from their original position. With several practice sessions most mothers can master manual expression. Once you have the motion down, rotate your fingers around the nipple to empty other milk sinuses.

When you begin expressing milk away from the baby, you will probably find that a few moments of gentle breast massage will stimulate the milk to let down. Catch the milk in any clean container. To get a greater amount, switch back and forth from one side to the other as soon as you notice the flow lessening. You can save time by expressing milk from both breasts at once, into containers on a table in front of you. Once you have learned how, the whole process should take about twenty minutes.

Using a breast pump In recent years breast pumps have become increasingly popular with nursing mothers. There are three basic types of pumps: hand- or foot-operated, inexpensive battery- or electric-operated, and hospital grade or near-hospital-grade. Since each pump has its own unique features, you will need to find the one that is best suited to your particular needs.

Hand- and foot-operated pumps. These pumps are portable and relatively inexpensive; the best are also comfortable and easy to use. They are ideal for at-home mothers who need to pump only occasionally. Listed as follows are the models most commonly available.

"Bicycle horn" pumps. These are available for less than ten dollars in some drugstores. A bulb is squeezed for suction, and the milk flows directly into it. Most authorities warn against using milk collected this way, since the bulb is difficult to clean and may harbor harmful bacteria. Many women find, moreover, that these pumps do not work well and can be uncomfortable. When used improperly, they can cause trauma to the breast or the nipple. And since they hold little milk, they must be emptied frequently.

▲ *bicycle horn pump*

Evenflo Comfort Care Manual Breast Pump. Available for about $20 in many drugstores and department stores, this pump creates suction by use of a plunger that is pulled outward.

Medela Little Hearts Breast Pump. This simple pump, operated by pushing and pulling the plunger, is available for about $23 from Medela pump rental stations and Medela, Inc., P.O. Box 660, McHenry, Illinois 60051. Call toll free 800-435-8316.

▲ *Evenflo Manual Pump*

Ameda One-Hand Breast Pump. With this pump you create suction by squeezing a hand grip. As the name implies, you can operate the pump with just one hand. The pump is available for about $33.50 from Ameda retailers and rental stations and from Hollister, Inc., 2000 Hollister Drive, Libertyville, Illinois 60048. Call toll free 877-992-6332.

▲ *Ameda One-Hand Pump*

Avent Isis Pump. A relatively new pump on the market, this one is becoming a favorite among nursing mothers. When you squeeze the handle, a soft silicone insert gently compresses the breast behind the nipple to stimulate milk flow. The Isis is available at baby-goods stores and from the manufacturer for about $40. To find a supplier or to order direct, write Avent America, Inc., 501 Lively Boulevard, Elk Grove Village, Illinois 60007, or call toll free 800-542-8368.

▲ *Avent Isis Pump*

First Years Easy Comfort Manual Breast Pump. This one is similar to the Avent Isis pump but has fewer parts and lacks the insert that massages the areola to stimulate milk flow. The milk flows into a bottle that can be used for feeding, and an extra bottle is provided. The pump sells for about $20 at department stores.

Medela Harmony Breast Pump. With a soft breast shield and a squeeze handle, this manual pump offers two basic settings for speed and vacuum strength, one to stimulate let-down and the other to use after the milk starts flowing. Speed and vacuum strength can be separately adjusted to suit individual preferences. The pump is available for about $45 from Medela pump rental stations and Medela, Inc., P.O. Box 660, McHenry, Illinois 60051. Call toll free 800-435-8316.

Gerber Manual Breast Pump. With a flexible silicone breast funnel, this pump is operated by squeezing the handle. The pump is available at drugstores and department stores for about $25.

Evenflo ComfortEase Manual Breast Pump. This squeeze-handle pump has adjustable suction and a silicone insert for more comfortable pumping. Available at drugstores and department stores for $22 to $30.

Cylinder pumps. Available in many drugstores and department stores as well as maternity shops, cylinder pumps used to be very popular with nursing mothers. They consist of two plastic cylinders. Suction is created by sliding the outer cylinder away from the breast, starting with short, frequent pulls to initiate the milk flow. If the head of the pump is not angled, the mother may need to lean slightly forward. After two or three ounces are collected, it is usually necessary to empty the milk into another container. Cylinder pumps range in price from about $25 to about $30. There are many brands on the market, but the following are tried and true:

▲ angled-head cylinder pump

- *Ameda Cylinder Breast Pump.* This angled-head pump is available from Hollister, Inc., 2000 Hollister Drive, Libertyville, Illinois 60048. Call toll free 877-992-6332.

- *Lansinoh Easy Express Breast Pump.* This straight-head pump is available in many drugstores and department stores. Call toll free 800-292-4794.

▲ straight-head cylinder pump

Medela PedalPump. This foot-operated pump may be less tiring to use than hand-operated models. And because it permits pumping both breasts at once, it may be the best choice for the mother who must regularly leave her baby but can't afford to rent or buy a fully automatic pump. The PedalPump is used with the Medela single- or double-pump kit (see "Hospital-Grade Pumps," page 183). The PedalPump sells for about $55, the double-pump kit for an additional $49. Both pump and kits are available from Medela rental stations and from Medela, Inc., P.O. Box 660, McHenry, Illinois 60051. Call toll free 800-435-8316.

▲ *Medela PedalPump*

Inexpensive electric pumps. Pumps in this category run on power from an electrical outlet, batteries, or, in some cases, either of these. Some of these pumps are semi-automatic; that is, the pump provides the suction, but the user must release it. Other pumps in this category are fully automatic. Fully automatic pumps remove milk more effectively than semi-automatic ones and are preferable especially for mothers who are routinely apart from their babies. Some of the fully automatic pumps in this category, however, cycle much more slowly than the 50 to 60 times per minutes ideal for stimulating let-down and emptying the breast completely. I recommend these pumps for women who are apart from their babies no more than 20 hours per week.

Gentle Expressions Pump. Made in Japan, this semi-automatic pump uses two AA batteries; an AC adapter can be purchased separately. The suction is released by pressing a small button on the side of the pump. The pump can be purchased from drugstores and discount stores for about $60 with an AC adapter and about $45 without. Call toll free 800-843-4429.

▲ *Gentle Expressions Pump*

Gerber Battery/Electric Breast Pump. This pump has a flexible silicone breast funnel and includes an AC adapter. As with other semi-automatic pumps, you release the suction by pressing a button. The pump is available at drugstores and department stores for about $55.

▲ *Gerber Battery/Electric Automatic Pump*

Nurture III Pump. The semi-automatic Nurture III is about the size of a small aquarium pump. It has variable suction strength, single or double pumping capability, and a two-year warranty. The basic model costs $120 plus $7.50 for shipping; a deluxe model, including a tote bag, a refreezable ice pack, extra bottles, and an instructional video, costs $160 plus $7.50 shipping. Order either model from Bailey Medical Engineering, 2216 Sunset Drive, Los Osos, California 93402. Call toll free 800-413-3216.

▲ *Nurture III Pump*

Medela Mini-Electric Pump. This battery-operated Swiss-made pump both sucks and releases automatically. It cycles 32 to 34 times per minute, less often than larger, hospital- or near-hospital-grade pumps. An AC adapter is included. The basic Mini-Electric pump costs about $95; a model that allows pumping both breasts at once costs about $160. Both are available through Medela pump rental stations and from Medela, Inc., P.O. Box 660, McHenry, Illinois, 60051; call toll free 800-435-8316. The double-pump model is also available at some department stores, where it is labeled as the Little Hearts Double Deluxe Pump.

▲ *Medela Mini-Electric Pump*

Medela Double-Ease Breast Pump. Ideal for women who are separated from their babies less than 24 hours a week, this pump cycles approximately 32 times per minute. Running off either C batteries or electricity from a wall socket, this pump allows you to express milk from one or both breasts at a time, and it comes in an attractive leather-like bag with an insulated area for milk storage and refreezable ice packs. The pump is available for about $200 from Medela rental stations and from Medela, Inc., P.O. Box 660, McHenry, Illinois 60051. Call toll free 800-435-8316.

Evenflo Comfort Select Auto-Cycling Breast Pump. Available with either a single- or double-pump kit, this fully automatic pump, powered by battery or AC adapter, cycles about 38 times per minute. It is available in drug and department stores for about $40 to $50.

▲ *Evenflo Comfort Select Auto-Cycling Pump*

The First Years Natural Comfort Single Electric/ Battery Breast Pump. Although it is fully automatic, this pump, with its slow cycling, is similar to other small battery-operated pumps. The pump sells in department stores for about $40.

The First Years Double Electric/Battery Breast Pump. This pump has adjustable suction strength but is semi-automatic; that is, the mother must repeatedly release the suction. Operable either with batteries or electricity from a wall plug, the pump can be used for expressing milk from one or

▲ First Years Natural Comfort Single Electric/Battery Pump

both breasts at a time. The double-pump assembly is somewhat cumbersome and may pose fitting problems depending on the size of the breasts and the distance between them. This pump sells for about $60 at department stores.

The First Years Double Electric/Battery Breast Pump. Packaged in an imitation-leather bag, this pump cycles automatically about 60 times a minute and has a 90-day warranty. The pump is available for about $90 at department stores.

The First Years Easy Comfort Double Electric/Battery Breast Pump. Designed to compete with Medela's Pump in Style (see "Near-Hospital-Grade Pumps"), this pump cycles 60 times a minute and comes with an imitation-leather bag, extra shields, and bottles. As with the other First Years pumps, the cumbersome double-pump assembly may pose difficulties for women with large or widely spaced breasts. The pump is warrantied for 90 days and is available at discount stores for about $150.

Whisper Wear Pump. This innovative, battery-powered pump allows a mother to express milk hands-free without removing her bra. The pump has automatic cycling, variable suction, and two speeds, one to stimulate let-down and one for expression. The milk drains into collection bags that are designed specifically for the pump and can be re-ordered as necessary. The pump uses AA batteries, which last about a

▲ Whisper Wear Pump

month, and is warrantied for one year. Two models are available: a single-pump model for about $120, and a double-pump model for about $220. They can be purchased from some lactation professionals and direct from Whisper Wear, 2221 Newmarket Parkway, Marietta, Georgia 30067. Call toll free 877-252-1326.

Near-hospital-grade pumps. This group includes the more expensive pumps sold for personal use and also small rental pumps. All near-hospital-grade pumps are fully automatic and have adjustable suction. They are most appropriate for mothers who are separated from their babies 20 to 40 hours per week; women who are exclusively pumping are better off with the more effective hospital-grade pumps, which have internal pistons. The WIC (Women, Infants, and Children) program lends near-hospital-grade pumps to some of its participants. (See page 241 for more information on the WIC program.)

Medela Lactina and Lactina Select Electric Pumps. Weighing just four pounds each, these rental pumps are ideal for the working mother who can't or prefers not to buy her own pump and is pumping no more than 40 hours per week. The Lactina Select has a variable speed control, which many mothers prefer. Both pumps can be used with single- or double-pump kits. In case you'll be pumping where no electric outlet is available, a

▲ *Medela Lactina Electric (016E) Pump*

battery pack and an adapter for a cigarette lighter are available separately. Long-term rental rates are about $30 to $60 per month. To locate a rental station near you, call Medela toll free at 800-TELL-YOU or visit the Web site at www.medela.com.

Medela Pump in Style. This very popular model was the first fully automatic pump offered for sale to nursing women. Ideal for the working mother who is away from her baby for 20 to 40 hours per week, the Pump in Style cycles quickly, up to 60 times per minute, and it allows the user to pump one or both breasts at a time and to vary the suction strength. The original Pump in Style weighs about 4 pounds and comes in an attractive leather-like shoulder bag; the Pump in Style Traveler is the same pump in a

▲ *Medela Pump in Style Professional Pump*

microfiber backpack. Recently, Medela has introduced the Pump in Style Advanced, which comes in a microfiber shoulder bag and uses a dual cycling pattern—rapid during the first two minutes to stimulate let-down, then slower and deeper for efficient expression. Each pump comes with a one-year warranty and a battery pack to use when no electric outlet is available. Because the standard nipple shields have rather small tunnels, you may need to order a kit with large shields if your nipples are as wide or wider than a nickel. The suggested retail price for Pump in Style original is $309.95, for Pump in Style Traveler $329.95, and for Pump in Style Advanced $349.99. These pumps are available from various retail stores, from Medela rental stations, and from Medela, Inc., P.O. Box 660, McHenry, Illinois 60015. Call Medela toll free at 800-435-8316, or check the Web site at www.medela.com.

Ameda Purely Yours Breast Pump. This was the second fully automatic pump developed for purchase by working mothers. With this pump you can control both the speed—up to 60 cycles per minute—and the strength of suction, and you can pump either one or both breasts at a time. When an electric outlet is unavailable, you can operate the pump using six AA batteries. Extra bottles, refreezable ice packs, and a one-year warranty are included, and a tote bag is optional. The Purely Yours pump is available for about $230 with the tote bag or $195 without it from Ameda retailers and rental stations and from Hollister, Inc., 2000 Hollister Drive, Libertyville, Illinois 60048. Call toll free 877-992-6332.

▲ *Ameda Purely Yours Pump*

Ameda Elite Pump. Intended for rental use, the fully automatic Elite weighs only seven pounds, and you can vary both the rate and the strength of its suction. In case you'll be pumping where there's no electric outlet, one model comes with a built-in battery pack. Long-term rental rates of $30 to $60 per month are available through most rental stations. To locate a rental station near you, call toll free 877-992-6332 or check the Web site at www.ameda.com.

▲ *Ameda Elite Pump*

Hospital-grade pumps. These have several advantages over most other pumps:

- They are all fully automatic.
- At 48 to 60 cycles per minute, they closely approximate the sucking action of a baby.

- They promote complete let-down of milk. They are in general more gentle and effective at draining the breasts.

- They allow for pumping either one or both breasts at a time. Double pumping can significantly cut the amount of time needed to empty both breasts and may stimulate greater milk production.

For all these reasons, hospital-grade pumps are the best choice for maintaining milk production when a woman is exclusively pumping or is away from her baby more than 40 hours per week.

These pumps generally are not marketed to consumers, but are available for rent for less than the cost of formula feeding. Long-term rental rates are even lower, and sometimes they are covered by insurance.

▲ *Hospital-grade Pump*

Hospital-grade pumps are also heavier than other pumps.

Medela Classic Electric Pump. A sturdy machine weighing over 20 pounds, this fully automatic pump is widely available through rental stations. When you rent the pump you must purchase a single- or double-pump kit, at a cost of $45 to $60. Most rental stations offer reduced rates for long-term rentals. To locate a rental station near you, call Medela toll free at 800-435-8316 or check the Web site at www.medela.com.

Medela Symphony Breast Pump. This newly introduced pump stimulates milk let-down with a rapid cycling pattern for the first two minutes of pumping, and then changes to a slower, deeper expression mode. Women report that Symphony is very comfortable compared with other hospital-grade pumps, and for some mothers this pumps speeds milk collection. Rental rates for Symphony

▲ *Medela Symphony Pump*

are higher than for most other rental pumps, about $70 per month. To locate a rental station near you, call Medela toll free at 800-435-8316 or check the Web site at www.medela.com.

Whittlestone Expresser and UniPulse Expresser. The fully automatic Whittlestone Expresser uses a constant vacuum; the pump pulsates during milk expression instead of releasing suction. Newly introduced, the UniPulse Expresser is similar to the Whittlestone Expresser but has a higher suction capability. Each of these pumps has a soft breast shield that massages the breast during pumping. For more information about either pump, call toll free 877-608-6455.

Ameda SMB and Lact-E Breast Pumps. These automatic pumps are heavy, hospital-grade machines; the SMB weights over 20 pounds, the Lact-E about 12 pounds. Although these pumps cost about a thousand dollars each to buy, they are widely available through rental stations for about $2.50 per day, or at a reduced rate of about $1.00 per day long-term. Single- or double-pump kits can be used with either pump. To locate a rental station near you, call toll free 877-992-6332 or check the Web site at www.ameda.com.

INTRODUCING A BOTTLE

Getting your baby used to a bottle is important if she will be fed by someone else while you are away at work or school. It is best to wait until she is three to four weeks old before introducing a bottle. By this time nursing should be well established, so the bottle will not interfere with the baby's interest in the breast. Some babies refuse the bottle if it is first offered much after they are one month old.

It is generally best if someone other than the mother bottle-feeds the baby. You can manually express or pump your milk instead of nursing, then have your partner or someone else feed the milk to the baby. Most infants will continue to accept a bottle if it is offered about twice a week. Offering a bottle periodically will also give you the opportunity to practice manual expression or become proficient with your pump.

If you have waited longer than a month and the baby refuses to take a bottle, be sure to have someone else try. Frequently a baby is more confused and upset by the bottle when her mother tries to persuade her. Trying to force the baby is upsetting for everyone and rarely successful. Some parents have succeeded by offering the bottle while walking with the baby. Hold the baby facing away from you and bounce her gently as you walk. Some babies dislike the taste of formula; try breast milk instead. Tasteless silicone nipples may be more readily accepted than rubber types. Recently I've been successful in getting babies to take a bottle fitted with the Avent Fast-Flow nipple or the Evenflo HealthFlow nipple. Another technique that has been successful for some mothers is to nurse the baby for just a few minutes, then unlatch the baby and slip the bottle into her mouth. If she objects, you can try again after a few minutes more.

◀ *A baby may more easily accept the bottle if you hold her facing outward and walk.*

The baby who refuses a bottle may do surprisingly well with an ordinary cup, particularly if she is about six months or older.

COLLECTING AND STORING YOUR MILK

Most mothers who will be manually expressing or pumping their milk while away feel more secure if they collect and store a backup supply of milk ahead of time. You can safely store breast milk in the freezer compartment of your refrigerator for up to three months. If you have access to a deep freezer (maintained at 0° F.), you can store it there for six months or longer.

If you plan to store your milk in the freezer compartment, collect it in clean plastic containers; you can use small plastic baby bottles or disposable plastic bottle liners. More durable plastic bags, designed for milk storage, are also available (see Appendix A, page 248). For storing milk in a deep freezer, hard plastic or glass bottles are preferable. Because the entire amount must be used once breast milk is thawed, you will want to store small amounts in each container to prevent waste. If you are not sure how much milk your baby will want at each feeding, put about 3 ounces in each bag or bottle. Leave some room at the top of the container to allow for the expansion that occurs with freezing. Secure bottle liners by twisting the tops, bending them over, and closing the ends with rubber bands or twist ties. Be sure to label each container with the date you collected the milk.

If you wish to add more milk to some that is already frozen, chill it first in the refrigerator for about half an hour to keep the top layer of frozen milk from defrosting.

Occasionally a mother finds that her expressed milk has an unpleasant smell or taste. Certain vitamin or mineral supplements can cause this; so can steroidal nasal sprays. In either case, the affected milk is harmless.

Breast milk can take on a soapy smell if the fat has broken down, freeing fatty acids. Apparently, some women have an excess of lipase, the enzyme that breaks down the fat in milk. Usually they notice the soapy smell after the milk has been refrigerated or frozen, but in some cases the smell develops immediately after expression. Most babies will take such milk without complaint, but the peculiar odor and taste can usually be lessened or eliminated either by chilling the milk before freezing it, or by putting it directly into the freezer, then thawing it in the refrigerator before warming it in a hot water bath. If these methods fail for you, you can inactivate the enzyme by scalding the milk on the stove—that is, by bringing the milk almost to a boil—and then immediately refrigerating or freezing it.

Frozen breast milk often takes on a yellow color. This does not mean that it has gone bad.

The best time to collect milk for storage depends on your baby's routine. You may need to pump after a few feedings each day if he

▶ You can use a fully automatic breast pump with a double-collection kit to pump breast milk more quickly and efficiently.

nurses frequently around the clock; you may get only an ounce or two each time. But if your baby sleeps for five or six hours at night, you may be able to collect a few ounces of milk just before you go to bed or early in the morning, depending on what time he begins his sleep stretch.

While you are collecting milk at home you are also becoming more proficient at hand expression or pumping. Occasionally a mother finds that the pump she has purchased does not work well for her. If this happens to you, be sure to review the manufacturer's instructions and check to see that all the parts are present and properly connected. Most pumps require some practice. If you are not happy with yours, though, try a different style.

When expressing your milk either by hand or with a pump, switch from one breast to the other as soon as the flow starts to diminish. This is the most effective way to stimulate more milk flow. Massaging the breasts just before and during expression encourages milk let-down and also increases milk flow.

A small proportion of women have trouble getting their milk to let down while they are pumping. A more efficient pump usually improves the situation; a fully automatic electric pump with double-pumping capability is best.

At work or school, you will need a time and a place to collect your milk. Almost any private place will do—an empty office; an unused room; or a women's lounge, locker room, or health center. Talk to your supervisor if you need to make special arrangements for regular or extended breaks from work. You may need to deduct the time from your usual hours or make it up at the end of the day.

You will also need a place to store your milk. Investigate whether a refrigerator is available. If there is no refrigerator, you can take a small cooler with refreezable plastic ice packs inside. Milk stays cold for several hours in these coolers, which are also handy for transporting milk home or to the caregiver's. Coolers specially made for storing and transporting breast milk are commercially available (see Appendix A, page 245).

When you pick up the baby at the caregiver's house, you can leave milk in the refrigerator for the next day. Fresh refrigerated milk is best for the baby, since it retains more antibodies than frozen milk. If the milk will not be used the following day, however, it should be labeled with the date and frozen.

You will want to thoroughly instruct whoever is caring for the baby on how the milk is to be stored and prepared. Specific written guidelines, like those that follow, are most helpful.

Refrigerated Milk
Use refrigerated milk within 72 hours. Take the milk out of the refrigerator just before using. Gradually, over 5 to 10 minutes, warm the milk to room temperature in a container of warm water. Do not warm the milk in a microwave or on the stove.

Frozen Milk
Use milk within three months if it has been stored in the freezer compartment of a refrigerator. Milk stored in a deep freezer is good for six months or longer. Always use the oldest milk first. Thaw the milk either in the refrigerator, where it can remain up to 24 hours, or in water just before feeding, gradually increasing the temperature to warm. Do not defrost the milk in a microwave or on the stove. Whatever milk the baby does not take must be discarded. Breast milk should not be refrozen.

Occasionally, some caregivers express concern about the safety of handling breast milk; they apparently fear that diseases might be transmitted through it. You can assure your caregiver that breast milk is not a "biohazardous material." The U.S. Centers for Disease Control and the Occupational Safety and Health Administration (OSHA) agree that people handling and feeding breast milk need not wear rubber gloves nor store the milk in a refrigerator where no other foods are kept.

BACK AT WORK

Once you are back at work, you will discover what routines work best for you, the baby, and your milk supply. Nursing twice in the morning before you leave the baby is ideal. Some mothers find that bringing the baby to bed with them, if she isn't already there, and nursing an hour or so before getting up works well. You can nurse again just before you leave home or when you get to the caregiver's house. While you are at work, try to express milk about as often as you would be nursing at home. This means at least two expression sessions if you will be gone a full eight hours—three is even better.

After work, you may want to nurse at the caregiver's house before going home. Many mothers find this provides a welcome opportunity to relax and talk with the caregiver about the baby's day. Encourage the caregiver to schedule the baby's feedings so that he will be ready to nurse as soon as you arrive. This generally means the baby should last be fed about two to three hours before you are expected.

When you are at home, of course, you will want to nurse as much as possible. Some mothers encourage their baby to nurse more frequently during the evening and night; they find this helps to keep their milk supply plentiful.

Some women find they are unable to express as much milk as they would like, especially after three to four months post partum. At this point you too may notice a drop in the amount you can pump, but this doesn't necessarily mean you can't meet your baby's needs. Many women overproduce in the first few months; after about four months, milk supply is determined by demand. If before you were pumping excess milk, you might now find yourself producing only as much as the baby drinks while you are away. This means your body has adjusted to the baby's needs. Normal milk production is about 1.5 ounces per hour, so if three hours have passed since you last pumped you should get about 4 to 5 ounces combined when you pump both breasts.

If your milk production is good, but your caregiver is running out of the milk you save, find out just how much milk your baby is taking while you're away. In general, a baby needs about 1.5 ounces per hour. If your baby is in day care for 11 hours, she needs about 18 ounces per day. If she is taking much more than this, she is being overfed.

If you think that your milk supply truly is too low, be sure that you are not using contraceptives containing estrogen and that you are not pregnant. Whatever health-care providers may tell you, combination birth-control pills and the vaginal ring with estrogen typically lessen milk production. The progesterone-only "mini-pill' is usually fine. Keep in mind that after six months post partum pregnancy can occur before menstruation resumes. Besides a reduced milk supply, other possible symptoms of pregnancy are sore breasts, nausea, and a fussier-than-usual baby.

If your periods have already resumed, you may notice a large dip in milk production lasting from just before your period starts until the day of your heaviest flow. Some lactation professionals report that taking 500 milligrams of calcium and 250 milligrams of magnesium per day for a few days usually helps to avoid the dip in production, although some women find they need 1,000 milligrams of calcium and 500 milligrams of magnesium during this part of their cycle.

To ensure ample milk production, use a good pump. For mothers who work 20 hours or more a week, I recommend fully automatic pumps, both rental models and the new types such as Pump in Style and Purely Yours. If you use a cheaper type of pump, it may work well enough at first and then lose some of its effectiveness, so that it no longer stimulates and drains the breast as well as before.

Give your pump a checkup to be sure it's working properly. Check the tubing, connections, and diaphragms. If the rubber diaphragms get small tears, the pump won't work as well.

Be sure the nipple shields fit you right. If the tunnels are too narrow, the flow of milk may be cut off when the suction causes your nipples to swell. Medela and Hollister (the maker of Ameda pumps) sell nipple shields in various sizes for their pumps.

Since pumping too slow or too fast can reduce the volume of milk expressed, you should pump so that the nipple is pulled and released about 50 times a minute. You may have to count the cycles, since most pumps don't have speed controls labeled as such.

If you're not sure whether your pump is draining your breasts completely, try pumping 15 to 20 minutes after a prior pumping. If you get much more than a half ounce, the collection kit, or even the pump itself, may be doing an inadequate job. Some women have good results only with internal-piston pumps—that is, the large rental models.

Long stretches without pumping or nursing are problematic for milk production. To maintain good production, make sure you nurse or double-pump (that is, pump both breasts at once) at least seven or eight times a day, and at least every three hours during daylight hours. Pumping and nursing sessions should be more or less evenly distributed during the baby's waking hours. If your baby sleeps a long, 8- to 12-hour stretch at night, pump in the late evening, just before you go to bed, or very early in the morning. Nursing right before leaving the baby and as soon as you return will help, too.

To stimulate increased milk production, you might try fenugreek capsules, which are available in health-food stores for around five to seven dollars per 100. Take two to three capsules three times a day. You'll probably notice an increase in your milk supply within one to three days, but you can take the capsules for longer, if you like; some women use fenugreek for weeks or months without any difficulties. Keep in mind that this remedy will be less effective if your breasts aren't completely drained at least seven times in 24 hours.

Even if you follow all the other measures, if you cannot express milk as often as necessary at work, you may find that the baby needs a supplement when you are away. This may be formula, but if the baby is at least four months old and seems ready for solids, you may want the caregiver to begin introducing them.

Some mothers leak milk while they are at work. You may need to wear thick pads in your bra; keep an extra supply of them with you.

Or try silicone nursing pads, which don't absorb milk but instead apply pressure to prevent leakage (see Appendix A, page 244). Some mothers prefer to use plastic breast shells to keep their clothes dry. Although they usually serve the purpose, these cups can also encourage further leaking. Finally, wearing printed blouses or keeping an extra jacket or sweater at work will help hide any wetness.

If you and your partner are both working, you may be too overwhelmed by chores to cuddle and enjoy the baby as much as you would like during your hours at home. Perhaps you can afford to pay someone to come every week or so to catch up on the housecleaning.

Combining nursing and working takes a great deal of time and energy. Aside from the responsibilities of your job, the baby, and the rest of your family, it is very important that you take time to care for yourself. Nursing mothers need to eat well. Although it may be tempting to skip breakfast or lunch, most women who do this find they have little energy to meet the many demands of the day. Get up a little earlier, if you must, to fix a nutritious breakfast. Bring snacks such as yogurt, cheese, nuts, and fruit to eat throughout the work day. Some mothers find brewer's yeast gives them an energy boost and helps keep up the milk supply. To avoid constipation and plugged milk ducts, you will also need to drink plenty of fluids while you are at work. Finally, rest is essential. Most working and nursing mothers find they must go to bed earlier every night than they once did. If you can, take an hour's nap just before dinner, and nap on your days at home with the baby.

THE REWARD PERIOD: 6
FROM TWO THROUGH
SIX MONTHS

Caring for Yourself
Making Love
Nursing Your Baby
Distractibility
Night Waking
Starting Solid Foods

The period between the baby's second and sixth months is exciting and rewarding. With the newborn stage behind, most mothers feel relaxed and confident. The baby is more predictable, his needs easier to interpret. By three months, his crying lessens considerably. Day by day, the baby becomes more sociable and attuned to the people and things around him. Still, nursings are an important part of his day, intervals for nurture and nourishment at the breast.

Caring for Yourself

During this time, I hope, you are beginning to feel more like your usual self. Napping whenever possible is still important, especially if your baby is waking at night for feedings or if your energy seems low. Your intake of food and drink continues to be essential to your overall well-being. Neglecting your need for fluids could lead to constipation and, possibly, recurrent plugged milk ducts. Skipping meals or substituting "empty-calorie" foods for more nutritious ones could result in fatigue and rapid weight loss. If you are overweight, limit your weight loss to one pound per week; crash dieting could decrease your milk supply. Most nursing mothers lose weight gradually without worrying about snacks or calories, whereas others find that eating three regular, satisfying meals and limiting high-calorie snacks and beverages, such as juices and soft drinks, helps them to achieve their weekly goal.

MAKING LOVE

After the birth of a baby most couples need time to readjust to each other sexually. You can probably resume intercourse by the sixth-week postpartum exam. In the meantime, you and your partner can enjoy physical loving such as cuddling, kissing, massage, and fondling. If your perineum feels fine and you want to have intercourse at three or four weeks post partum, there is no reason to wait. But you may not yet feel ready even when your doctor, nurse, or midwife gives you the go-ahead.

You may be worried that intercourse will be painful. If you have had an episiotomy, you may feel some initial tenderness and tightness, but your stitches should be completely healed after one month. Relaxing as much as possible will help make lovemaking more comfortable the first few times. A warm bath, a glass of wine, and extra time with foreplay may be helpful. Be sure to use a generous amount of lubricating gel, such as K-Y Lubricant, Astroglide, or a contraceptive gel, in and around your vagina. You may also want to experiment with different positions, especially if you have had an episiotomy. Some women prefer to be on top so that they control the degree of penetration. Others find that a side-lying position feels best at first.

Most new mothers experience some vaginal dryness during love-making because of the hormonal changes that occur after giving birth. The vaginal secretions increase once regular ovulation resumes. Ovulation is generally delayed during nursing, for a variable period. Until your periods resume, a water-soluble lubricant can make intercourse more comfortable and pleasurable. I don't recommend creams containing estrogen, which when absorbed through the vagina can diminish milk production.

The breasts need not be off limits when making love. Some women, however, find them less sensitive to stimulation during the nursing period; they may also feel tender during the early weeks, and later on just after nursing. Breast stimulation and orgasm may cause the milk to let down and leak or spray. If leaking milk is bothersome for you or your partner, you might nurse shortly before you make love, or wear a blouse, a bra, or a nightgown during lovemaking.

For some time after having a baby, many women find they have less interest in making love than formerly. There are a variety of reasons for this. Estrogen, which influences a woman's sex drive as well as the amount of vaginal secretions, is produced in lower levels after she gives birth. Sometimes having so much skin-to-skin contact with the baby all day dampens a woman's desire for more physical contact.

A new mother may also fear another pregnancy—whether or not the recent one was planned. At the end of the day, too, a mother may be just too tired for lovemaking.

New fathers also suffer from overwork and night wakings. Like their partners, they may be too exhausted to make love, and they may also worry about having another baby too soon.

It is important that your intimacy as a couple continues. As with most other changes in life, talking over your feelings and making some adjustments will make this period easier.

Finding the time to make love can be difficult, especially when you are tired. You may need to plan times to be together when you are rested and when the baby is likely to be asleep. Making love early in the morning or when the baby is napping may work the best. Perhaps you can take a nap in the afternoon so you will have more energy for your partner in the evening. Having the baby sleep in another room may help you to feel more comfortable.

But if neither you nor your partner is much inclined to have frequent intercourse, don't feel there is something wrong with you—your physical and emotional intimacy can continue without it. Passionate feelings will probably come easier as the baby gets older. Remember, you have a lifetime ahead of you to share your love.

Contraception

If you are concerned about the possibility of getting pregnant again, talk over birth-control options with your partner and your health-care provider. Foam, condoms, IUDs, diaphragms, cervical caps, and surgical sterilization are all considered safe during nursing. (If you used a diaphragm or cervical cap before your pregnancy, you will need a refitting now.)

Many women want reliable and convenient birth control in hormonal form. Although "the pill" and other hormonal birth-control products apparently do no direct harm to the nursing baby, pills containing estrogen, even in low doses, often reduce a mother's milk supply and may thereby lead to poor weight gain in the baby. The vaginal ring (NuvaRing), the contraceptive patch (OrthoEvra), and one hormonal injection product (Lunelle) also contain estrogen and so can diminish milk production. These products are best avoided during breastfeeding.

Fortunately, not all types of hormonal birth control interfere with milk production. The progestin-only pill, also known as the "mini-pill," has no effect on milk supply. Nor do progestin-only injections, which give three months protection against pregnancy, or Norplant subdermal implants. All of these products are considered safe during breastfeeding.

Whichever birth-control method you use, its reliability is increased by the fact that you are breastfeeding. For now, in fact, breastfeeding may be the only birth-control method you need. That breastfeeding affects fertility is a truth that has been largely ignored in a century when partial breastfeeding and early weaning have been the norm. But breastfeeding has provided more contraception world-wide than all other methods combined. Frequent nursing, especially during the first several months after birth, suppresses ovulation in most women. If a woman hasn't yet had a period, in fact, exclusive breastfeeding provides her more than 98 percent protection against pregnancy in the first six months post partum (Kennedy, 1989). But when her periods resume, when the baby is receiving any food or drink besides breast milk, or when the baby reaches six months of age, the mother's chance of getting pregnant again increases. If you want to rely on breastfeeding-as-contraception (which medical texts call the Lactational Amenorrhea Method, or LAM), nurse at least eight times in every 24 hours, with no more than six hours between nursings and a cumulative sucking time of at least 60 minutes per day. For best results, don't feed formula or solids or even use pacifiers.

Once your periods resume, you may prefer to track your natural menstrual cycle, abstaining from intercourse around the time of ovulation instead of relying on birth-control pills or devices. If you want to use the "rhythm method," try to get personal instruction in it. Learn to keep track of all three basic body measures: basal body temperature, cervical mucus, and length of menstrual cycle.

NURSING YOUR BABY

As your baby quickly grows and develops you will notice her nursing pattern also changes. You can expect two more appetite spurts during this period, the first at about two and a half to three months and the second between four and a half and six months. As with the earlier appetite spurts, the baby will nurse more frequently for a few days to stimulate an increase in milk production. Most mothers produce 30 to 36 ounces of milk or more each day during this period, a 50 to 80 percent increase over the first month.

By three or four months of age, many babies have dropped a feed-
; or two and are nursing about seven or eight times a day. Nursing
less often than seven times a day may result in decreased milk production and slowed weight gain for the baby. This most commonly
occurs when a baby spends much of her day sucking on her fingers or
on a pacifier, or when she begins sleeping long stretches at night but
isn't nursed more often during the day. It can also happen when a
working mother expresses milk infrequently while she is away. Your
baby should continue gaining an ounce a day until she is three to four
months old. Between three and six months of age, a breastfed baby
normally gains one-half ounce or more each day.

During this period, some women begin to fear that their babies
aren't "getting enough." You may find that your breasts feel less full,
that you leak less or not at all, and that the sensations of the milk letting down are less intense than before. None of this necessarily means
your supply is low or your baby isn't getting enough milk. If your
baby is taking the breast at least seven times in 24 hours, has plenty
of wet diapers and has yellow bowel movements, and seems content
after feedings, you probably have no reason for concern. Your breasts
may feel less full simply because they have adjusted to your baby's
needs and now produce only as much milk as she wants.

However, if your baby does not suck well or take the breast often
enough, if you are using a birth-control product containing estrogen,
or if you are taking a medication that can interfere with milk production (such as a decongestant like Sudafed or an antihistamine like
Benadryl), your production may truly be low. The baby's weight gain
is the best gauge of adequate milk production. A quick weight check
at the doctor's office may help you feel more confident.

Some babies prefer to nurse from just one breast at each feeding.
So long as the baby seems content and is continuing to gain enough
weight, this is normal.

You may also notice that your baby is nursing for shorter periods.
She can now get a large quantity of milk quickly because both she
and your breasts have become so efficient.

Most three- to six-month-old babies are chubby; some may be
quite plump. Parents and sometimes even doctors may become concerned about the baby who gains weight above the norm. These
babies slow their growth during the second half of the first year and
typically begin to slim down during toddlerhood. It is not advisable
to restrict the baby's nursing because of her weight.

DISTRACTIBILITY

Between three and five months, a baby starts to become more aware of the world around her. When she can see clearly across the room and interact more with her family, she goes through a phase of becoming easily distracted while nursing. At any new, sudden, or interesting sight or sound, she pulls away from the breast to look around. Older siblings are a common distraction. At around this age the baby may also start to play nursing games; she may stop sucking, for instance, to pat Mom's face and smile. Although these antics can be adorable, you may become frustrated if nursing sessions become longer and longer because the baby seems never to want to get down to the "business" of nursing.

This behavior does not mean the baby has lost interest in nursing. Of course, you'll want to rule out any contributing problem, such as a low milk supply or painful reflux. But if the baby is generally content, you needn't worry about her distractibility. It may help to nurse while lying down in a quiet, semi-darkened room. Some mothers reserve for nursing sessions a special toy—a blanket or necklace that the baby likes to hold and stroke—to keep her from being distracted by other things.

After several weeks of interrupted feedings, your baby will no longer have to let go of the nipple to check out what's going on around her. Instead, she'll turn her head with the nipple still in her mouth.

NIGHT WAKING

Although some babies start sleeping in stretches of up to 10 hours as early as six weeks of age, most continue to wake at night until they are six to twelve months or older. Most babies, especially those under six months of age, can be expected to wake up to nurse at least once each night, and as often as every three hours.

Night wakings may frustrate you, especially if your older child or a friend's baby slept long stretches at an early age. If you are tempted to give the baby formula or cereal in a bottle just before bedtime in the hope of encouraging him to "sleep through," keep in mind that night waking is normal for a baby this age. Besides, as many studies have shown, feeding cereal early has no effect on when a baby starts sleeping through the night. Sleeping patterns are affected by many things, including temperament.

Babies who sleep long stretches during the first few months typi-
ʟally begin waking again around three to four months of age. Perhaps
teething is to blame. Other signs of teething may include general fussiness, drooling, changes in nursing patterns, biting, and finger sucking.
Giving the baby a cold washcloth or a chilled water-filled teething ring
to bite on may make her more comfortable. Some doctors recommend
the use of gum gels and acetaminophen drops (such as Infants' Tylenol
or Tempra) for teething pain. A baby may also wake more at night
when daytime nursings decline, because Mom is away during the day,
because he gets distracted during daytime feedings, or because he
spends too much time sucking his finger or a pacifier. To encourage
your baby to get more of his milk during the day and evening, try
offering the breast in a quiet, darkened room, nurse whenever he
begins sucking his fingers, and limit the use of a pacifier.

Waking every one to two hours all night long is *not* normal for a
baby this age. If your baby starts waking very frequently, perhaps
teething, an ear infection, or another illness is to blame. If he has recently
had a cold or an ear infection, his ears may be the problem now, even if
he has no fever and isn't pulling on them. If the baby has never been a
good sleeper, reflux or a low milk supply might be causing the problem.
For more information, see "Fussiness, Colic, and Reflux," page 152.

If your baby wakes frequently at night, for whatever reason,
taking him into your bed for all or part of the night may make nursing easier and lessen your own sleep disruptions. For information on
bed sharing, see "Sleeping with Your Baby," page 129.

For additional information on babies and sleep, I recommend the
book *The No-Cry Sleep Solution* by Elizabeth Pantley.

STARTING SOLID FOODS

Probably no area of infant development attracts as much confusion
and range of opinion as the starting of solid foods. Your family,
friends, and child-care advisors probably all have different ideas on
when and how to begin giving solid foods to your baby. By far the
most sensible approach I have found is that of Ellyn Satter, a nutritionist who breastfed her own three children. I highly recommend her
book *Child of Mine: Feeding with Love and Good Sense* (1991).

Solid foods are best introduced when a baby becomes developmentally ready for them and is able to benefit from the nutrition they
offer. Although this does not happen until a baby is close to six
months of age, many mothers feel pressured to begin solids earlier.

Some think of feeding solids as a sort of status symbol, something to brag about. But the American Academy of Pediatrics now recommends that breastfed babies not be fed solid foods until they are at least six months old.

You'll know your baby is developmentally ready for solid foods when he can sit with support, control his head and neck movements, and tell you he is hungry or full by leaning forward with an open mouth or pulling away and turning his head. He may indicate his readiness for solids by grabbing food off your plate or out of your hand.

At this time he will also begin to lose his tongue-thrust reflex, which causes him to push anything in his mouth forward and out. This means he will be better able to eat from a spoon, move the food to the back of his mouth, and swallow. The baby's digestive system will also be mature enough to handle solids at this time. His kidneys will be able to excrete the waste products of solid foods, and he will be less likely to develop allergic reactions from them. His iron stores will lessen, so the iron from solid foods will be beneficial for him.

Offering solids prematurely means replacing breast milk, which is nutritionally perfect, with foods that are nutritionally incomplete. Additionally, the early introduction of solids may lead to obesity (perhaps lifelong), allergic reactions, decreased milk production, and early weaning. Rest assured, your milk provides all the nutrients your baby needs for at least the first four to six months after birth. Besides, holding off on solids is practical: The closer to six months you introduce them, the more likely you will be able to skip the "baby food" stage and start with table foods.

CONCERNS
ABOUT YOURSELF

Recurrent Plugged Ducts and
  Breast Infections
Overabundant Milk

CONCERNS
ABOUT THE BABY

Slow Weight Gain
One-Sided Nursing
Sudden Refusal to Nurse

CONCERNS ABOUT YOURSELF

Recurrent plugged ducts and breast infections

Many nursing mothers experience recurrent plugged ducts or breast infections. If you are suffering from either at the moment, carefully review the information in "Survival Guide: The First Two Months," pages 140–144. If you have had more than two or three episodes, the following suggestions may be helpful in preventing more.

Treatment Measures for Recurrent Plugged Ducts and Breast Infections

1. Be sure that you are nursing the baby frequently, and that at least one breast is emptied well at each feeding. Avoid skipping or delaying feedings. To encourage complete drainage of the milk ducts, massage your breasts gently while nursing. Pick a quiet place to nurse if your baby gets distracted during feedings. Wake the baby at night if your breasts feel too full. If your baby routinely sleeps for long periods at night, consider using an effective breast pump before you go to bed, after the first morning feeding, or both. This way you'll ensure that your breasts are completely drained at least once or twice a day.
2. Change nursing pads whenever they become wet.
3. Get as much rest as possible. Nap whenever you can. Consider sleeping with the baby if you aren't already.
4. Make sure you are getting plenty to drink every day.
5. Check your bra and any other restrictive clothing you may be wearing.
6. If your doctor prescribes antibiotics, take the entire course. A ten-day prescription may be needed; a five- or seven-day course may be insufficient for complete treatment.
7. If an infection recurs in the same part of the breast shortly after antibiotic therapy has ended, the antibiotic may be ineffective. Some antibiotics do not penetrate breast tissue as well as others. Discuss this possibility with your doctor or pharmacist.
8. Take a daily iron supplement if you are anemic.
9. Many lactation professionals believe vitamin C supplements may help prevent recurrences of breast infections. Some suggest that taking supplemental lecithin (three capsules a day) and avoiding saturated fats in the diet may prevent plugged milk ducts.

10. A high salt intake may increase susceptibility to breast infections. Some women seem to be prone to breast infections premenstrually; this may have to do with the fact that they retain water just before their periods. If your periods have resumed, try limiting your salt intake for several days before your period is due.

11. If a plugged duct or breast infection does not go away within three days, consult a physician.

Overabundant milk

Some mothers continue to be bothered by an oversupply of milk after two months post partum. You are not necessarily producing too much milk, however, if you leak or become engorged during the baby's long sleep stretches. Only if you are still feeling uncomfortably engorged most of the time should you consider taking steps to decrease your milk supply.

Treatment Measures for an Overabundance of Milk

1. Continue drinking plenty of fluids. Decreasing fluids does not decrease milk production.

2. Nurse your baby at just one breast per feeding. Let him suck as long as he likes on one side. If you become uncomfortable, express a small amount of milk from the other breast. Switch breasts with each feeding.

3. Should you be caught in a routine of expressing milk while nursing full time, gradually decrease the amount of milk you take until you are no longer expressing any.

CONCERNS ABOUT THE BABY

Slow weight gain

A two- to three-month-old baby is considered a slow gainer when he is putting on less than an ounce a day. A slow-gaining three- to six-month-old is gaining less than one-half ounce per day.

A baby who is discovered to be gaining weight slowly, not gaining at all, or losing weight may be nursing too infrequently—that is, fewer than seven times in a 24-hour period. Between three and four months of age, most babies find their fingers or become avid pacifier users. Some babies stop letting their mothers know when they are hungry and instead suck away at fingers or a pacifier, decreasing the number of nursings to fewer than seven a day. The baby who sleeps eight or more hours at a stretch each night may fail to get enough milk if he doesn't nurse at least seven times during his waking hours. A baby may also slow his weight gain after losing some interest in nursing because juices or solid foods have been introduced prematurely, especially if they have replaced nursings.

Slow weight gain may occur, too, when a working mother fails to express her milk often enough while she is away from the baby, causing an overall decrease in her milk supply. Estrogen-containing birth-control pills, even the low-dose kind, often decrease milk production. Occasionally, a baby who has never had normal weight gain suddenly becomes a worry to his physician and parents. This happens because health professionals do not always identify a newborn who gains less than an ounce a day during the early weeks as being underfed. Eventually such a baby may become obviously underweight. This is sad, since a low milk intake can be much more easily remedied if the problem is recognized early on. A milk supply that has been low for two, three, or even four months can be very difficult to improve.

Treatment Measures for Slow Weight Gain

1. Devote at least two to three days to nursing the baby and doing little else. Put the pacifier aside, and each time you notice the baby beginning to suck a finger offer the breast. You may find yourself nursing every hour or so, although increasing feedings to eight or more per 24 hours is usually sufficient to quickly increase milk production. If your baby is sleeping through the night, try to include at least one late evening feeding. You might also consider waking the baby for a feeding after he has slept five or six hours.

2. While the baby is nursing, listen for swallowing. As soon as you notice the swallowing taper off, switch breasts. Continue switching back and forth for as long as the baby is willing to continue, ideally at least 10 minutes. If the baby is easily distracted, nurse in a quiet, darkened room.

3. If your baby has been losing weight or has never gained weight adequately, consider giving him supplemental formula while you work on increasing your milk supply. For instructions on estimating the amount of milk you are producing and the amount of milk your baby needs, see "Underfeeding," page 162.

4. Consider taking fenugreek capsules and perhaps even a milk-stimulating medication to help increase your milk production (see pages 78–80).

5. Should your baby refuse to nurse as often as every two hours or resist switching back and forth, you might consider expressing or pumping milk after each nursing to stimulate an increase in milk production. An electric pump may be most convenient. After two or three days of this regime, both the baby's nursing pattern and your milk supply should begin to improve.

6. If you are working, try to spend two or more consecutive days at home following the recommendations just given. While you are at work, express milk as often as possible. If you cannot express milk often enough, you may need to supplement with formula on days you are with the baby.

7. After two or three days of stepped-up nursing, you should notice that your breasts feel fuller and that the baby swallows over a longer period during feedings. Continue nursing frequently, at least eight times a day. Have the baby's weight checked after a week of frequent nursing, and again a week after that. If the baby still isn't gaining well, supplementation with an ounce or two of formula after some of the feedings may be necessary. You can add cereal to his diet, once or twice daily *after* nursing, if the baby is four months or older.

One-sided nursing

Occasionally a baby develops a preference for one breast over the other. Perhaps the favored breast produces more milk or lets it down more rapidly. Sometimes there is no apparent reason—the baby simply prefers one side. Twins usually choose opposite sides.

Sometimes a mother unknowingly nurses the baby more at one breast than the other, increasing milk production on the favored side. Some mothers prefer nursing on one side only; in certain cultures one-sided nursing is common.

One breast can fully support a baby's nutritional needs. But if a single baby nurses substantially more at one breast than at the other, the less used breast may become noticeably smaller. After weaning, the breasts will equal out in size.

Treatment Measures for One-Sided Nursing

1. Offer the baby her least favorite side first. After she has nursed on both sides, encourage her to nurse on the first side again.

2. Should the baby totally refuse one side, try changing positions. Use the football hold, or nurse while lying on your

side. The baby may be more willing when she is sleepy or actually asleep, or when you nurse in a darkened room.

3. Increase the milk supply in the less used breast by manually expressing or pumping milk after each nursing for a few days.

4. If all else fails, simply accept your baby's preference to be a one-sided nurser.

Sudden refusal to nurse

Occasionally a baby under six months suddenly refuses to nurse. A "nursing strike" usually lasts for a few days, but sometimes for as long as two weeks. It rarely means the baby is ready to wean. Weaning seldom occurs this suddenly. See "Nursing Strike" (page 226) for the reasons behind this problem and suggestions for coping with it.

If your baby suddenly refuses one breast but is happy to nurse at the other, see "One-Sided Nursing," page 207.

NURSING THE 7 OLDER BABY

Caring for Yourself

Nursing Your Six- to Twelve-Month-Old

Coping with Teething

The Transition to Table Food

As breastfeeding progresses to six months and beyond, the nursing relationship continues to change. Although the baby is busy exploring the world around him and has probably shortened most of his nursings, breast milk continues to be his primary source of nutrients until he is well established on table foods. Breastfeeding also continues to provide protective antibodies against illness.

For you, nursing provides the opportunity to sit down for a few minutes and just enjoy your baby. Nursing may also become your main tool to help your baby fall off to sleep at naptime and bedtime.

CARING FOR YOURSELF

You may sometimes feel tired and run-down during your baby's second half-year. Becoming more active and getting overtired seems to be especially common around six months post partum. Certainly, eating poorly and losing too much weight can contribute to a loss of energy. Taking it a bit easier, getting some extra rest, and paying attention to your diet can do a lot to improve your overall well-being. Taking brewer's yeast or a B-complex preparation may also be helpful.

Resuming your periods

If your periods haven't resumed yet, they may well do so during your baby's second half year. Although some women see the resumption of their monthly cycles as early as six weeks after birth, most women's periods resume as their babies begin eating regular meals at the table. Other women, especially those who nurse frequently, don't

start menstruating until 12 to 24 months post partum. Y
periods may be lighter, heavier, or less regular than norma.

In most cases, fertility returns before menstruation. If you don
want to become pregnant again soon, you should be using some form
of birth control even if your periods haven't resumed.

Both nursing mothers and their babies may feel out of sorts
around the time of menstruation. Some mothers report that their
babies fuss for a couple of days, or even refuse to nurse for a short
time, when periods resume. Other women experience sore nipples for
a few days between ovulation and the start of menstruation.

Often, a nursing mother experiences a dip in the milk supply a
few days before her period starts. Although this dip tends to be greatest during the first few cycles, some women have milk-supply problems at the time of their periods for as long as they continue nursing.
Calcium and magnesium supplements may help; try taking 1000
milligrams calcium and 500 milligrams of magnesium each day just
before and during your period. If your periods are very regular, you
can also try taking fenugreek capsules in the few days before you
expect your period to start (see "Underfeeding and Weight Loss,"
page 76).

Nursing Your
Six- to Twelve-Month-Old

The typical baby of this age is venturing out on his own and seemingly
becoming more independent, but he often scampers back to the safety
and reassurance of his mother's arms. By eight to ten months, in fact,
he probably cannot bear to have his mother out of his sight for even a
minute. This is known as separation anxiety. Until the baby learns to
trust that his mother will return, out of sight means gone forever.

During the first six months, both babies and their mothers tend
to be captivated by nursing; they give it all their attention. After the
first four months, babies are easily distracted; if anything catches
their interest they may pull off the breast momentarily. As your baby
passes six months and develops more motor skills, he may still be
somewhat distractible, and he will probably become more active
during nursings. This is a normal stage of development and a healthy
part of the nursing relationship. Your baby may play with his foot
and smile at you as he nurses. He may adopt some really annoying
behaviors—pinching the breast, pulling or twiddling the nipple, or
doing acrobatics while nursing. You can put an end to these antics by

holding your baby's hand or giving him something else to hold—a beaded necklace, for instance, or a soft blanket.

Between six and twelve months, you should be nursing your baby seven times a day, on average, and feeding him solids only after nursing. Some people might tell you that four nursings a day are sufficient, but this number is normal only for formula-fed babies, who take more at a feeding and tend to eat more solids than breastfed babies of the same age. You may also hear that you should expect your baby to go longer between daytime feedings. In fact, as your baby begins to sleep longer stretches at night, he may need to nurse more frequently during the day—as often as every two hours—to get as much breast milk as he needs.

Crawling and cruising babies can be so busy that they may not "ask" to nurse as often as they should. If your baby goes longer than three hours during the day without expressing a desire to nurse, take him to a quiet, dark room and offer your breast, or put on a brightly colored scarf or beaded necklace before picking him up. Some mothers reserve a special toy just for nursing sessions.

At around seven to nine months of age, many babies go through a stage in which they seem to lose interest in nursing. The parents may be told that their babies are "self-weaning." In truth, babies rarely wean themselves without cause before one year of age, and most babies will happily nurse for two to four years without initiating weaning. In most cases of "self-weaning" in seven- to nine-month-old babies, what actually happens is a nursing strike (see pages 226–227). Usually, the baby's normal distractibility results in infrequent nursing, which in turn causes a low milk supply. If the mother takes measures to rebuild her supply, the baby will happily return to nursing. Even if the milk supply is abundant, it's best to assume that when a baby under 12 months loses interest in nursing he does so because of a problem that can be corrected. Teething pain, a sore throat, a stuffy nose, and an ear infection are all possible reasons that an older baby might temporarily refuse to nurse.

Many women notice that it takes longer for their milk to let down in the second six months of nursing. This may be a sign of a dwindling milk supply. Delayed let-down may contribute to a baby's loss of interest in the breast, especially at about nine to ten months of age.

Many parents and physicians worry when weight gain in a healthy breastfed baby dramatically slows in the second six months after birth. Keep in mind that most U.S. babies are totally weaned to formula and solids by six months of age, and that formula-fed babies tend to gain more weight between six and twelve months than breastfed babies. The charts used in most doctors' offices reflect this unnatural growth pattern. Normal weight gain for a breastfed baby between six and twelve months is 1 to 4 ounces per week. Babies with small parents fall in the lower end of this range.

Night wakings are another common concern during a baby's second half-year. Some older babies sleep from bedtime until dawn, but most wake more often. Parents of a six- to twelve-month-old baby who is still waking at night may get a great deal of conflicting advice. Well-meaning family members may say that night waking is not normal. Pediatricians may point out that a baby this age does not "need" to nurse at night. Still, waking one to three times a night is entirely normal for babies as old as two years, and some six- to twelve-month-olds may actually wake to nurse at night out of thirst or hunger.

A baby's night wakings can be handled in a variety of ways. Some mothers find that sleeping with their babies disrupts their own sleep less, while others prefer to get up, nurse, and return the baby to a crib. If a baby wakes very frequently, it's best to figure out why. Teething, an ear infection, separation anxiety, stomach problems, an allergy, a chill from kicking off the covers, or a low milk supply are all possible causes.

Coping with Teething

By six months of age, most babies begin teething. This can affect their nursing patterns. Some babies are less interested in nursing when their gums are tender, and others want to nurse more often, especially in the night. To soothe your baby's aching gums, give him things to munch on during the day, such as a cold, damp washcloth or a teething ring. You might freeze and slightly thaw the washcloth or teething ring before offering it to him. If he fusses during nursing sessions, you can rub his gums with a cold washcloth or apply Baby Orajel just before nursing. If your baby is very uncomfortable, acetaminophen or ibuprofen may help (see "Survival Guide: Months Six through Twelve," page 224).

Many mothers worry that the eruption of teeth means that nursing must come to an end. But babies and toddlers with teeth can and usually do nurse without causing pain to their mothers' nipples. While the baby is sucking, the tongue protects you by covering the lower teeth. In other words, so long as a baby is swallowing milk, she cannot bite. If your baby does bite you, you can take measures to make sure it doesn't happen again (see "Biting," page 222).

Some mothers find that their nipples get sore during teething even though their babies aren't actually biting. When babies are cutting teeth, they may adjust their latch on the breast to put pressure on sore areas of their gums. This can make the nipples sore. To avoid the problem, ease the baby's pain before nursing with one or more of the remedies I've just described. If you feel tenderness while nursing, adjust the baby's position at the breast.

Once your baby has teeth, you need to know how to keep them healthy. "Baby-bottle tooth decay," the major cause of dental caries in toddlers and preschoolers, results when the sugar in milk, juice, and other beverages feed bacteria that produce acid, which erodes tooth enamel (the acid in juices, if they are allowed to pool in the mouth, erode the enamel directly, too). This condition is especially common in babies and young children who are put to bed with a bottle. Even if your baby never drinks from a bottle, tooth decay can occur. To prevent this, gently wipe your baby's first teeth with a gauze pad after feedings and at bedtime. You can try using a soft toothbrush once your baby has seven to eight teeth. Wet the toothbrush, but don't use toothpaste. Fluoride toothpastes are not recommended until a child is three years old.

The Transition to Table Food

A baby shows readiness for solids when he sits up, reaches for food at the table, and generally acts interested in eating what his family eats. Although a baby may do these things at five months or so, it's generally best to put off giving solids until the baby is six months old, when his digestive system is more likely to be nutritionally ready for them.

From six to eight months When your baby is close to six months old, you may begin to notice that he still seems hungry after nursing. If after a few days of stepped-up nursings he still seems unsatisfied, feel free to experiment with solids. Occasionally a four- to five-month-old fails to gain sufficient weight, or stops gaining at all. If normal weight gain doesn't resume after a week or so of more frequent nursings, it may be time to begin solids.

Quite a variety of foods have been recommended as the solids for infants: fruits, vegetables, meats, yogurt, egg yolks, cottage cheese. But all of these foods contain either too much carbohydrate, protein, or fat, or too little iron.

An iron-fortified baby cereal mixed with breast milk is the ideal first solid food for a baby. It meets both his nutritional and his developmental needs. Cereal meets the baby's increased demand for iron that occurs around six months. Mixing the cereal with milk provides a good proportion of carbohydrate, protein, and fat. The texture of cereal can be adjusted to match the baby's ability with semisoft food.

Rice or barley cereal is less likely to cause an allergic reaction than wheat or a mixed-grain cereal, and is therefore a better first food (be sure to check the label, as some rice cereals do contain other grains). Although they are sometimes recommended for infants, cereals that must be cooked do not contain as much iron as dry baby cereals, and what iron they do contain is not nearly as well absorbed. Ready-made baby cereals in jars also have less iron than the dry versions, and are more expensive. High-protein cereals provide more protein than young infants need.

Mix dry baby cereal with breast milk, formula, or evaporated milk diluted one to one with water. You can use whole cow's milk (less than eight ounces a day) if your baby is six months or older and you are not concerned about an allergic response. Breast milk or a hypoallergenic formula (soy-based or "predigested") is probably the best choice if you are concerned about allergies. Mixing the cereal with water or juice will not provide protein and fat for the baby.

Nurse your baby before offering cereal or another solid food. It is important to do this until he is eating three regular meals of table food, at some time after eight months of age. Until then, breast milk will continue to be his most important food.

Begin with one feeding of cereal a day. At first, mix one teaspoon of cereal with enough milk to make a thin paste. At the first few feedings, don't be surprised if your baby pushes back out almost as much as you have put in. It may take a little time before he learns to move the food to the back of his mouth and then swallow it. Should your baby become upset and refuse to eat, wait a few days before trying again.

Gradually increase the amount of cereal you give at each feeding, and add a second feeding so the baby is getting a total of one-half cup of mixed cereal a day. Thicken the mixture as his eating ability improves. If you are giving supplemental iron, stop when the baby is taking one-third to one-half cup of mixed cereal a day.

Sometime after her sixth month, when your baby is taking a total of a half cup of cereal in two feedings a day, she is ready for other foods. She should still nurse before eating, however, until she is well established on table foods and is having three meals a day. The nutrients in breast milk are the ones that she needs most.

Because fruits and vegetables offer vitamins A and C, they become important in the baby's diet as her intake of breast milk drops. They also accustom her to different tastes and textures and encourage the development of tongue control and chewing ability. Although puréed fruits and vegetables, whether commercially prepared or homemade, are nutritionally adequate, they do not accustom the baby to different textures or help her learn chewing skills. Commercial baby food in jars may be appropriate when you are eating out or traveling, but at other times mashed soft fruits and vegetables are best.

The order in which fruits and vegetables are introduced isn't all that important. Some nutritionists and others feel that vegetables may be more readily accepted if they are introduced before fruits, whose sweeter flavor many babies prefer. Fresh or canned fruits can be mashed, scraped, diced, or chunked according to your baby's ability. Fresh or frozen cooked vegetables are preferable to those that are commercially canned, as these usually contain too much salt for a baby. A food mill or baby-food grinder can be handy for vegetables that are hard or stringy. Offer only one new food at a time, waiting a few days before introducing another. In this way, should a certain food upset the baby, you will have a good idea which one it is.

A meal pattern that works well during this transition time is cereal and fruit in the morning and cereal and vegetables in the evening. Use a fresh or frozen vegetable from your own dinner before it is salted or seasoned.

Although one to two tablespoons of fruit is adequate, babies usually like the taste so much they are eager for more. Limit the baby to one-quarter or one-third cup per serving; too much fruit can cause intestinal upsets and diarrhea.

You can offer fruit juice instead, but limit the amount to three ounces a day. "Juice abuse" is a common mistake in infant feeding. Not only do babies not need more than three ounces, but juice often lessens their appetite for milk and solid foods. Overdependence on juice can lead to diarrhea and, especially when given in a bottle, to tooth decay. Avoid "fruit drinks," which contain mostly water, some juice, and sugar. Be careful with citrus, tomato, and pineapple juices—they can cause allergic reactions in some babies. Rashes, wheezing, nasal stuffiness, and diarrhea may be allergy symptoms.

Juices bottled for infants are expensive and unnecessary. Once opened, fruit juices should not be stored in metal cans.

Juices are probably best offered from a cup. Most babies are ready to begin learning how to drink from a cup by the time they are seven or eight months old. At first you will need to hold the cup for the baby. Once she begins holding her own cup, be prepared for her turning the cup over to see what happens—all a part of the learning process. You can try a training cup, which comes with a tight-fitting lid and a spout and therefore won't spill; however, some babies suck from these, so the lesson goes unlearned.

One or two tablespoons of vegetable is sufficient for the baby. Vegetables high in nitrates, such as beets, carrots, and spinach, should be limited to this amount. When young infants are given excessive amounts of these vegetables, the nitrate can convert to nitrite in their bodies. This can cause the displacement of oxygen in the blood, leading to fast breathing and lethargy. *Methemoglobinemia*, as this condition is called, becomes less of a possibility after the baby is six months old and has more acid in her stomach.

Dark green and orange vegetables, such as broccoli, carrots, sweet potatoes, and squash, should be given no more than three or four times a week. Given too often, they can cause the baby's skin to turn yellow. This is completely harmless, however.

During this time you can also offer the baby breads and dry cereals. These offer B vitamins and iron. Although the baby may not actually eat much at first, she will be developing her chewing and self-feeding skills. Rice cakes and dry Rice Chex or Corn Chex are good first choices before trying wheat-based breads and cereals. The chance of an allergic reaction to wheat lessens once the baby is seven or eight months old, but you may want to put off offering wheat even longer if anyone in the family is allergic to it.

Try not to worry should your baby eat very little before she is eight months old. She will have her own food preferences, and she may refuse a certain food one week and happily eat it the next. She may refuse all foods for a while if she is not feeling well. And, as she becomes interested in feeding herself, she may also turn her head away from any food offered from a spoon. Although she'll be messy, you should let her feed herself. Give her another spoon, or allow her to use her fingers. Let her examine her food before deciding whether or not to eat it. By feeding herself, your baby will develop her grasping skills and hand-eye coordination. Be patient if she plays with her food instead of eating it; keep in mind that your breast milk is still the most important part of her diet.

From eight to ten months

Probably at some time between eight and ten months of age, your baby will become interested in what the rest of the family is eating. Again, I take my recommendations from Ellyn Satter and her wonderful guide to infant and toddler feeding, *Child of Mine: Feeding with Love and Good Sense* (1991).

Once table foods are offered, three major transitions follow. The first is adding another meal or two so the baby is eating three or four times a day. The second is adding high-protein foods—such as meat, poultry, fish, shell beans and lentils, eggs, cheese, and tofu—as the baby's intake of breast milk drops. The last transition is postponing breastfeeding until after the meal; this encourages the baby to take more solids.

This new meal pattern basically requires the addition of a midday meal and, perhaps, a small snack. Continuing to give a half cup of fortified infant cereal over one or two meals (or a meal and snack) is still important. Two servings of bread, at one-quarter slice a serving, complete the baby's requirement for grains. At least four daily servings of fruits and vegetables, at one or two tablespoons a serving, are recommended. Juice may substitute for one serving but should still be limited to three ounces a day.

The baby also needs at least two servings of high-protein foods every day. A serving of meat, poultry, fish, or eggs is about one tablespoon, or one-half ounce. Although chicken and fish (carefully boned) are fairly easy for the baby to manage, red meats may need to be shredded, ground, or minced. Avoid lunch meats and hot dogs, which are high in salt and nitrates and are not the best sources of protein. The baby can have an egg three or four times a week. Should allergies be a concern, cook the egg until solid and offer only the yolk. Other high-protein foods for a baby of this age include: 1 ounce of hard cheese, 1/4 cup of cottage cheese, and 1/2 cup of shell beans or lentils. Commercially prepared "infant dinners" are a poor source of protein, being mostly vegetables and water with only a small amount of meat.

Should you prefer that your child have a vegetarian diet, this is easy so long as cheese and eggs are included. Do take the time to learn all you can about vegetarianism and the nutritional needs of infants and toddlers; *Child of Mine* and *The New Laurel's Kitchen* (see "Suggested Supplemental Reading," page 297) will get you started. You might also want to consult with a nutritionist, especially if you are considering a "vegan" (vegetable-only) diet. Young children on such diets are at substantial risk for B-vitamin deficiencies and, because of a lack of protein, general growth deficiencies. The federal Women, Infants, and Children (WIC) nutrition program or your local public health department can probably refer you to a nutritionist who can offer further guidance.

While your baby may not always get precisely the suggested amounts of grains, fruits, vegetables, and high-protein food every day, averaging close to these amounts over a week will ensure he is well nourished. But if by eight to ten months your baby will still take solids only sporadically at best, it may be time to give him a little extra encouragement. If his growth curve falls off, and, perhaps, he seems to be sick a lot, he may be becoming too emotionally dependent on the breast, and substituting nursing for eating a variety of nutritious foods. In this case, make sure you are nursing after meals, not before. If he is desperate for the breast, try to keep the nursing short, then encourage him to return his attention to other foods. Always include him in family meals, but offer food at other times of the day if he refuses it at mealtimes. If he resents your pushing solids, have someone else feed him or let him feed himself. Never assume that because he spits something out in disgust one day he won't take it a week later.

From ten to twelve months   After the baby is established on table foods, the final transition is adding milk along with the meal. Ideally this should be accomplished when the baby is between nine and twelve months of age. Whole milk is more digestible now that the baby is eating table foods. Low-fat milk is not a good choice because it does not provide the fat that the older baby or toddler needs. Evaporated milk, diluted one to one with water, can be used, however; this may be more convenient if the rest of your family drinks low-fat milk. Because evaporated milk is treated with high heat, it is more digestible than whole milk, and it is no more expensive. You can use soy formula or another hypoallergenic formula if your baby is allergic to milk. If your baby does not like milk of any sort, offer plenty of cheese and yogurt, and try tofu—it is also very high in calcium.

The baby's fluoride supplements should be stopped now if your water is fluoridated to 0.3 parts per million.

You may be wondering if we have just weaned your baby. In a sense, yes. Weaning is the *process* of expanding a baby's diet to include other foods. For another year or two or more, however, nursing may continue to be important and convenient for early morning feedings, snacks, naps, bedtime, and general soothing and comforting.

Biting
Night Waking
Nursing Strike
Considering Weaning
Weaning the Older Baby

BITING

Being bitten by a baby while nursing is a common yet unforgettable experience. A baby most commonly bites before her teeth come in, often just before the top two teeth break through. Your baby may bite your breast because she is biting everything and anything that relieves the ache in her gums.

Your baby is most likely to bite at the end of a feeding or when she is just snacking; she may have a playful look on her face and may push the nipple to the front of her mouth just before she takes a chomp. This behavior may continue for several days, but it usually ends as suddenly as it began.

Some mothers fear their babies will start biting once the first teeth have come in. This occasionally happens, but it is usually because other areas of the gums are sore, and not because the baby wants to try out her new incisors. When a baby bites, the usual advice is to say NO loudly, and then not to nurse for at least 30 minutes after the bite. This doesn't work with all babies, however; some get so frightened that they go on a nursing strike. Others enjoy the reaction and want to continue the game. I recommend the following measures instead.

Coping Measures for Biting

1. Avoid letting the baby snack at the breast during this period of biting.
2. Just before feedings, offer the baby a cold, damp washcloth or a chilled water-filled teething ring.
3. While you're nursing, keep your finger ready to end the feeding. Watch for a change in your baby's nursing pattern; as soon as she stops taking long even sucks and begins short choppy ones, end the feeding. If you notice a playful look on her face, end the feeding.
4. If the baby has your nipple between her teeth, pull her in close to your breast to partially block her nose; she'll release the breast to breathe. Many persistent biters give up when they realize that biting triggers this uncomfortable position.
5. If you resume nursing and the baby tries to bite again, she is obviously not hungry any more. End the feeding.

NIGHT WAKING

Although some older babies and toddlers sleep well at night, many wake frequently, night after night. Your baby may in fact be waking more at night and napping less during the day than she did in the first few months. You may have thought that when your baby reached six months or older and started taking solid food that his nighttime wakings would diminish. You probably even know someone whose baby "sleeps through the night." But such a baby is atypical. When health professionals talk about sleeping through the night, they are referring to a six-hour stretch. Although some babies sleep a six-hour stretch, most breastfed babies wake two or more times a night. Many babies who slept long stretches in the early months wake more frequently later.

You may think something is wrong if your baby doesn't sleep through the night. You may wonder if she wakes because of teething, illness, hunger, thirst, digestive problems, wet diapers, chilling or overheating, superior intelligence, upcoming developmental milestones, or separation anxiety. Although any of these might perhaps contribute to night waking, the basic cause may simply be your baby's need for a snack and a cuddle.

As you may suspect, breastfed babies are less likely to sleep through the night. Chances are your friend's sleeping baby is already weaned or was never nursed at all. One study found that whereas weaned babies slept a median of nine to ten hours at a stretch at every age after four months, nursing babies slept in bouts of four to seven hours to the end of the second year (Elias et al., 1986).

Not only do breastfed babies sleep in shorter bouts than do bottle-fed babies, but nursing babies also sleep less overall. In the Elias study, weaned babies slept a median of thirteen to fourteen hours throughout the first two years, but nursing babies gradually lessened their total hours of sleep from a median of fourteen to a median of eleven hours.

Why do bottle-fed babies sleep in longer stretches than breastfed babies? Marsha Walker (1993), a lactation consultant, points out that babies formula-fed from birth have poor "vagal nerve tone"; that is, their autonomic nervous systems are measurably disordered. This makes them sleepier and less alert than breastfed newborns. Poor vagal tone in a newborn, by the way, is related to inferior motor and mental development for at least two years after birth.

Babies who are weaned after several months of breastfeeding may start sleeping through the night for other reasons. They certainly have waking episodes, as everyone does, but these babies fall back into deep sleep without any intervention from parents. Most have probably learned to go back to sleep alone—through the use of a thumb, pacifier, or bottle, through their parents' ignoring them, or perhaps with a sophisticated method such as scheduled awakenings, whereby a parent arouses a child in time to prevent spontaneous awakenings, until both spontaneous and scheduled awakenings are gradually eliminated. In most of these cases, the parents' desire for separation has overcome the baby's natural urge to be close to other human beings.

No one knows for sure why weaned children sleep more overall than those who are still nursing. It seems babies often nurse during light sleep; they release the nipple when they fall into deep sleep. This may be why a child who was obviously tired will, instead of falling asleep after a long nursing, wake up seeming completely refreshed. If nursing in a light-sleep state were counted as sleep, the average total hours of sleep might not vary at all between nursing and weaned children.

Whether or not you've identified a reason for night waking, you may be spending a considerable amount of energy trying to end it. Manipulating daytime naps, feeding solids late in the evening, giving pain relievers or cold remedies when the baby isn't sick or in pain, trying to keep the baby from falling asleep at the breast, consulting health-care providers, and trying different tactics in the middle of the night rarely work.

This is not to say that you shouldn't have your baby examined if you suspect a physical discomfort. She could be hurting from an ear infection (especially if she has had a runny nose in the past couple of weeks) or from teeth working their way in. Some babies who are distracted during many of their daytime nursings may wake often at night out of hunger.

If your baby seems to be waking from severe teething pain, you can try giving her acetaminophen (such as Baby Tylenol) or ibuprofen (such as Baby Advil). Of the two, ibuprofen seems more effective for teething pain. If one of these medications wears off before it's time to give another dose, you can "piggyback" the two pain relievers— that is, give the other in the meantime. Call a pediatric nurse for more detailed advice.

Offering pacifiers, bottles, or other comfort objects in the night is not likely to get you a full night's sleep. Most parents who try these things must get up at night to find them when their babies wake up crying. Besides, unless a bottle is filled with water, a baby risks developing tooth decay when she falls asleep at night drinking from one.

One way some parents succeed at making a baby sleep through the night is by letting her "cry it out" for a few nights or more. Several books tout this technique, perhaps the best known among them being Richard Ferber's *Solve Your Child's Sleep Problems: The Complete Practical Guide for Parents* (1985). The idea is to refuse to pick up your baby when she wakes during the night, but to let her cry herself back to sleep, until she learns that her crying is fruitless. Although this may seem drastic, many parents report that it has worked for them.

If you decide to try this strategy, choose a three- to four-day period in advance. When your baby wakes crying, go to her every five minutes. Lay her down; say, "It's night-night time"; and leave. Most babies cry up to an hour or so the first night, and for a shorter time the next two or three nights. If this technique solves your night-waking problem, you can still continue nursing during the day.

A kinder way of training babies to sleep through the night is advocated by Elizabeth Pantley, a mother of four and the author of *The No-Cry Sleep Solution*. The no-cry method involves early, long naps, before-bed routines, and early bedtimes. Nighttime wakings are handled this way: As soon as the baby cries, you nurse her back to sleep. Over time, you gradually shorten the baby's time at the breast, with the aim of ending the nursing as soon as she stops actively sucking, before she is fully asleep (you must stay awake yourself, of course, to manage this). When the baby can fall back to sleep without extended sucking, you comfort her when she wakes just by patting her on the back and repeating a soothing word. Eventually, the baby should be able to go back to sleep on her own with just a word. If the baby shares your bed, you may want to help her stay asleep by holding her hand against your breast. Pantley's book includes sleep charts for tracking the baby's progress.

After developing her method with her own children, Pantley tested it on 60 other mother-baby pairs. More than half of the mothers had their babies sleeping through the night within three weeks, according to Pantley, and 92 percent succeeded within two months.

If Pantley's and Ferber's methods fail to work for you, you might consider the way nursing mothers all over the world have made night waking less disruptive: Sleep with your baby. Despite what people say, your baby won't be smothered by the covers or by your or your mate's shifting body. The baby won't keep you awake; babies with easy access to the breast rarely cry at night. After a few nights you'll adjust to the new sleeping companion, and her presence will not disrupt your sleep as much as would waking to her cries, getting out of bed, tending to her, and coming back to bed again. Neither you nor your baby will need to waken completely to nurse, and Dad won't need to waken at all.

If taking a baby into the parents' bed puts a damper on sexual activity, couples who have adopted this approach seldom complain about a lack of sex. Parents do mention how much they enjoy watching their baby sleep, cuddling her warm little body, and waking up with her in the morning.

Families have come up with many inventive ways to make the "family bed" more comfortable, safe, and convenient. You might buy a larger mattress, build a platform for mattresses placed side by side, or simply put your mattress on the floor. So your mattress stays dry, get a waterproof mattress pad; so *you* stay dry, double-diaper the baby or consider using disposables at bedtime. This will eliminate most nighttime diaper changes; when you or your mate must get up, a low-wattage nightlight will make things easier.

If you have doubts about sleeping with your baby, you might still try it for a couple of weeks before dismissing the idea. You can find more detailed advice on bed sharing in Tine Thevenin's *The Family Bed: An Age Old Concept in Child Rearing* (see page 298).

If you're still feeling worn out after you've found some way to get more sleep at night, you might examine your diet. Some lactating women may be vulnerable to fatigue because of vitamin B deficiencies. Although in such a case the baby will generally grow well and get the nutrients she needs from her mother's milk, her mother may suffer from low energy levels. Be sure you are eating plenty of whole grains, which are rich in B vitamins.

You might also consider supplementing your diet with brewer's yeast, a potent source of B vitamins that is considered more effective and faster-acting than B-complex supplements. Available in health-food stores, brewer's yeast can be taken as a tablet or as a powder to be mixed with juice or milk. Starting with the daily dose recommended on the label, you can slowly increase the amount to two to four times the daily recommendation (increasing the amount too quickly could cause diarrhea in you and your baby).

NURSING STRIKE

Although nursing strikes can occur at any time, they usually happen in the second half of the baby's first year. A nursing strike is distinguished from weaning by its suddenness. Some babies wean themselves between eight and twelve months of age, but they usually do so gradually.

Reasons for nursing strikes vary greatly. They may include teething, a cold, an ear infection, a painful herpes sore in the mouth, or a change in the taste of the milk. They sometimes happen after a prolonged separation between a baby and his mother, or after a baby has bitten his mother and been frightened by her response. Sometimes, when a baby has become used to a bottle and its rapid flow of milk, his refusal to nurse is a response to his mother's dwindling milk supply. Some authorities believe a nursing strike may precede mastery of a major motor skill, such as crawling, standing, or walking.

Although some mothers decide to turn a nursing strike into final weaning, in most cases the baby can be coaxed to resume nursing. Strikes typically last a few days, but they may go on for as long as two weeks.

Treatment Measures for Nursing Strikes

1. Try a change in position, or nurse in a quiet, darkened room.
2. So long as the baby refuses to nurse, pump or manually express your milk frequently throughout the day. Offer the milk in a cup rather than a bottle.
3. Try to determine the cause for the nursing strike. Consider having the baby examined to rule out an ear infection or other physical problem. Check your milk supply, especially if the baby has been nursing infrequently or has become increasingly dependent on a bottle: Do your breasts feel empty most of the time? Is the milk slow to let down? Is the baby swallowing less?
4. Maintain frequent and close skin-to-skin contact with the baby without nursing. Offer the breast whenever the baby is sleepy.

CONSIDERING WEANING

For any of various reasons, you may be considering giving up nursing altogether. If you truly resent breastfeeding, if you need to give it up because of a serious illness, or if you are planning to get pregnant soon, you can wean completely and easily at this stage (see "Weaning the Older Baby," page 229).

Perhaps the reasons you want to stop nursing are less compelling. Maybe months ago you set a time limit for breastfeeding and now you feel you must carry through with your plan, or maybe you think your baby is simply too old to nurse. You may have heard a myth—that older babies all bite or that weaning a toddler is just too difficult.

Or you may hope that ending breastfeeding will solve various problems like the shape of your body, fatigue, marital troubles, or sibling rivalry. Rarely does total weaning solve problems like these. Many women who end the breastfeeding relationship early later regret that they have given up this precious time for no benefit.

It is normal to feel ambivalent about nursing. Sometimes you may wish you could be free of this intense relationship, and other times you may adore putting your baby to your breast and watching him fall off to sleep there. Such ambivalence is a natural part of an intimate relationship. Simply recognizing this may help put your mind at ease.

Perhaps the problem is friends and relatives. If they have started asking when you plan to wean the baby, you may feel embarrassed and pressured to give up nursing. Our society seems to rush babies and toddlers to independence. Keep in mind that nursing is still providing your baby with protective antibodies; even at twelve months, a baby has only 60 percent of an adult's ability to fight off infection. If a friend's baby weaned early and easily, remember that some babies need the comfort of the breast much longer than others. Babies who are allowed to wean themselves do so when they feel that their source of security will always be there when they need it.

Since your nursing older baby will soon be a talking nursing older baby, you might consider what word you'll feel comfortable hearing your baby use in public for breastfeeding. Words like *booby* might be fine at home, but they could cause you embarrassment elsewhere. You might choose a term such as *nursie* or *numnums* or use a word that your baby makes up.

If this doesn't keep friends and relatives from making comments, you may decide to ignore the comments, confront the people who make them, or keep your nursing a secret from them. You won't, of course, be able to hide your nursing relationship from your partner, whose comments may be the hardest to deal with. If he is bothered by your breastfeeding, you can try telling him about its benefits to your baby's health and to your family's finances. If your baby is waking at night, you might invite your partner to take over night duty.

You can find support for your continued nursing by seeking out mother-to-mother support groups such as La Leche League. See Appendix A, page 240, to learn how to locate a local group.

Weaning the Older Baby

Weaning the older baby need not be hard, especially if she is crawling and busily exploring or has lost interest in some of her nursings. Ideally, weaning at any age should occur gradually, over several weeks at least. A good place to begin is with the nursing that the baby seems least interested in, most likely one during the day. Key to your success is providing an appealing substitute for the breast. This means offering not only something else to eat or drink, but also yourself. Nursing provides a mother's love and attention as well as food. You'll need to do a lot of cuddling and rocking, and activities like reading a book or playing on the floor together.

You must choose whether to wean to a cup or a bottle. Although the older baby is developmentally ready for a cup, if she has trouble swallowing from one, the bottle may be best. However, giving the baby a bottle can lead to other difficulties. If she is not carefully monitored, she can become overdependent on the bottle, lose interest in solid foods, and end up with serious tooth decay. If you wean the baby to a bottle, of course, you will probably need to wean her *from* it later on.

Unless the baby is well established on table foods and eating three meals a day, give formula before offering solid foods.

Although weaning may progress quickly for some babies, concluding in a month or two, other babies take longer, especially those who are especially fond of nursing or are reluctant to give up certain feedings. The first nursing in the morning and those before nap time and bedtime are often most loved by the older baby. It may take longer to eliminate these completely. For helpful advice, read *The Nursing Mother's Guide to Weaning* (see "Suggested Supplemental Reading," page 298).

8 NURSING THE TODDLER

Nursing during Pregnancy
Tandem Nursing
Your Toddler's Diet
Weaning Your Toddler

The toddler is trying to accomplish the major task of establishing himself as an individual. Although he is no longer a baby, he is still very dependent. One minute he is exploring and getting into everything, and the next he is turning to his mother for comfort and reassurance.

Many toddlers tend to nurse briefly. Some nurse just a few times a day, but many want the breast often. Moreover, a toddler may nurse a few times one day, and many times the next. Even if he nurses infrequently, the antibodies in breast milk are still present and protective. The breast is important to the toddler not only for a quick snack and help in falling off to sleep, but for intermittent comfort and emotional refueling. Sometimes nursing is one of the toddler's few connections to a busy mother.

You may discover that nursing into toddlerhood is not only a convenient way of mothering, but that it is one of the few times during the day that your child holds still long enough for cuddling and affection.

Some nursing toddlers still wake at night for feedings. See "Night Waking" (page 223) for suggestions and coping strategies.

The young toddler may be quite insistent when he wants to nurse, regardless of the time or place. As he gets a bit older he will become more willing to wait a little while.

Children in many parts of the world are breastfed until they are two, three, or four years of age, yet nursing a walking, talking toddler is considered somewhat deviant in parts of Western society. Many toddlers are dependent on a bottle, pacifier, thumb, or blanket, and this is quite accepted, but a mother who is nursing a toddler may have to deal with veiled or point-blank suggestions that her child is too old for it. The concerns about nursing beyond infancy often reflect the fear that a child will become spoiled or overdependent. In fact, when a toddler's need for security is met, he becomes more self-assured and independent.

Mothers who are nursing toddlers usually enjoy socializing with others who are doing the same. La Leche League is not only supportive of women who breastfeed beyond the first year, but also offers meetings for those who are nursing young children. (See Appendix A, page 240, for more information on La Leche.) Norma Jane Bumgarner's book *Mothering Your Nursing Toddler* (1982) is an excellent resource for those nursing beyond infancy (see "Suggested Supplemental Reading," page 297).

Nursing during Pregnancy

Although many people frown on breastfeeding during pregnancy, there is no reason you cannot continue nursing your child when you find out another is on the way. Fears that nursing will lead to miscarriage or a malnourished newborn have no basis, even for mothers who are too queasy to eat much. Whether to wean is best left up to you—but if your child is less than a year old, it may be best to delay weaning at least until he is regularly eating solid foods and drinking from a cup.

Pregnancy often causes a decrease in milk supply. If your baby is much less than a year old and you notice your milk supply declining, you may need to supplement your milk with formula. Some nursing babies and toddlers wean themselves during their mothers' pregnancies. Others do not seem to mind the changes in the milk and show no signs of wanting to give up nursing.

Many women who nurse while pregnant experience tender breasts and sore nipples. These are due to the hormonal changes of pregnancy. Although this soreness usually goes away as the pregnancy progresses, there is no known cure for this problem except weaning. Many women also feel especially tired at first—this again is a normal response to pregnancy. Plenty of rest helps combat fatigue, especially in the first trimester.

Some pregnant mothers may notice uterine contractions while nursing. No studies have shown that such contractions lead to premature labor, but if you have had a previous premature labor you should discuss this possibility with your doctor.

In the second and third trimesters, an excellent diet is essential for the nursing mother.

Tandem Nursing

Mothers who have nursed throughout all or most of their pregnancies may find themselves nursing an older baby or toddler along with the new baby. This may be overwhelming for some, particularly if the older child is nursing frequently. But many have found it to be a generally positive experience.

Because the breasts are receiving more stimulation than if the mother were nursing only one, the milk is usually plentiful. As a rule, the younger baby should be nursed first. Bumgarner's *Mothering Your Nursing Toddler* (1982) includes a detailed section on tandem nursing (see "Suggested Supplemental Reading," page 297).

Your Toddler's Diet

Toddlers are notorious as sporadic eaters. Their appetite decreases during this time—first because their growth slows down tremendously from that of the first year, and second because they are often too busy to eat. The toddler grows more in length than in weight. Weight gain typically slows to a pound or less every two months.

The toddler's feeding skills vary considerably. Sometimes she may feed herself, and other times she wants to be fed. Parents who worry about how little their child eats may be tempted to persuade, trick, or even force her to eat more. This turns meals into battles and may be the start of long-term feeding problems. As Ellyn Satter says, "You are responsible for *what* your child is offered to eat, *where* and *when* it is presented. She is responsible for *how much* of it she eats."

The suggested minimum servings of foods for the toddler are similar to those for the older baby. A handy rule of thumb is this: Give one tablespoon per year of age or one-quarter of the adult serving, whichever is easiest to figure for the particular food. You would therefore offer your toddler two tablespoons of peas or one-quarter of an apple. The suggested daily minimum servings for each food group are as follows:

- Fruits and vegetables: 4 servings
- Grains (bread, cereal, noodles, rice): 4 servings
- High-protein foods: 2 servings
- Milk: 2 to 3 cups

Offering a meal or nutritious snack every three to four hours is a good approach with a toddler. Don't always offer milk just because she likes it; if she drinks more than three cups a day it may replace other nutritious foods in her diet. Expect that your toddler may enjoy a certain food one day and refuse it the next. Make sure she comes to the table for meals and is offered whatever foods the family is eating. Do not play into her food whims by running out to the kitchen to fix something else for her when she refuses to eat.

WEANING YOUR TODDLER

Ideally, complete weaning occurs when both the child and the mother are ready for it. Many times, though, a mother begins to think about weaning while her toddler is still happily nursing. She may feel that weaning will make things easier—that it will put an end to night waking, make the baby more independent, or improve her own energy level. Some mothers have a self-imposed deadline for weaning and begin to feel pressured once it draws near. Others simply become fearful that their children will nurse forever if allowed. Most often, a mother considers weaning when other people suggest that the baby should no longer need to nurse. Criticism from friends, family, or health-care workers may be straightforward or subtle, but it often motivates a mother to end the nursing relationship.

All mothers have mixed feelings about nursing at times. Keep in mind that weaning will not help your child sleep through the night, improve your relationship with your partner, make you less tired or less bored, or make your child less dependent on you. Toddlers, especially, often demand to nurse more when their mothers become busier and when they receive little mothering except at the breast. At times that young children need more attention, ironically, mothers often feel most like they need some kind of a break. Weaning during these times can be terribly upsetting for a child, and for the rest of the family as well. Should the arbitrary date you had in mind for weaning arrive, there is no need to follow through if you and your child are still enjoying nursing.

Knowing all this, you may still have trouble dealing with the disapproval of friends and family members. Families in particular can wield tremendous influence over a nursing relationship. You may be able to deal with criticism from others by either ignoring it or confronting it. Or you may choose to withdraw from those who are critical and find new friends who believe in nursing older babies; a mother-to-mother support group, such as La Leche League or the Nursing Mothers Counsel, is one place to do this. Finally, you might simply keep your nursing secret from those who don't approve.

When a baby is still nursing often and enthusiastically at the end of his first year, he will probably want to continue nursing throughout the second year and beyond. Some experts say a child rarely initiates weaning before the age of four. For this reason friends may tell you to wean by your baby's first birthday if you have definite feelings against nursing a three-year-old. You may fear that, if you wait, you will have a major struggle convincing your child to stop nursing in the months to follow. That toddlers seldom initiate weaning, however, doesn't mean they always fight it. Should you find yourself still happily nursing at your baby's first birthday, be assured that there will probably be several opportune times to wean and numerous techniques to accomplish weaning after a year of age and before the age of four.

You might rightly initiate weaning if you have definite feelings against nursing a toddler or nursing while pregnant. Weaning—or simply limiting the number of daily feedings—may also be best if you are starting to resent nursing. The decision to wean should be made carefully, not in reaction to a bad day or a temporary problem.

Timing is important once you've decided to wean. Keep in mind that weaning is a process rather than an event. Weaning initiated by the mother should ideally occur gradually and empathetically over several weeks, at least. And there are better times than others to initiate the process. If the child is particularly clingy and needy, if he has recently had a stressful experience such as moving or starting child care, or if you are actively trying to get him to sleep through the night, now is not the time to wean.

Some specific suggestions for weaning can be found under "Weaning the Older Baby," page 229. (For further advice, read *The*

Nursing Mother's Guide to Weaning (see "Suggested Supplemental Reading," page 298). In general, mother-led weaning involves substituting for nursing something that the child enjoys as much. In this way weaning does not become a series of deprivations or rejections. If the pace of weaning is too rapid, most children will react with obvious unhappiness or increased dependency on a pacifier, a thumb, or a bottle. Occasionally weaning must be postponed for a few weeks because the child is simply unable to cope without nursing.

Unfortunately, no one technique works for every mother and toddler. The best recommendations involve finding substitutions and distractions that may satisfy the child, while at the same time ensuring that his needs for food, love, and attention are met. No plan is likely to succeed, however, unless a mother is sure of her own desire to wean. Her attitude is most important to her success.

Before you begin, pay close attention to the child's nursing routine, and yours. Keeping a record for a few days, like the one below, may give you some valuable insights for developing an effective plan.

Time	Place	Interest level	Reason for nursing
5:30 pm	*kitchen*	*high*	*hunger*

Take note of when and where you nurse, the child's level of interest in nursing, and what you think prompted his demand for the breast. From the toddler's point of view, nursing may be just the thing whenever he is bored, frustrated, or tired, or he wants your attention or comfort—as well as when he is hungry.

From your observations, you should be able to identify which nursings are least crucial to your toddler and get some clues as to what type of substitutions will most likely satisfy him. Some nursings may be easily replaced with a nutritious snack or something to drink. Substitutions for toddlers may include any number of activities— playing with a special toy, reading a book, taking a walk, or visiting with another toddler. Warm-weather months may be an easier time to encourage weaning, as most toddlers enjoy exploring out of doors.

Although you may be able to substitute certain predictable daily nursings with other activities, if your toddler nurses sporadically all day you may sometimes need to coax him to postpone nursings. Delaying daytime nursings works well for some toddlers as long as some distraction is provided. This can be an effective way to further weaning.

Some of your nursings are probably associated with routines the two of you have established, and with recurrent situations in which your toddler wants to nurse to get your attention. Identify these instances so you can change the pattern. If you nurse in bed early in the morning, get up instead—get dressed and offer your child breakfast. If you have a favorite place to relax and nurse, stay away from it. If your toddler demands to nurse every time you talk on the phone, keep conversations short. If you sit in front of the television and nurse, do something else or he will want to continue with the usual pattern. Think creatively of ways your child can learn new routines.

You can also take advantage of your child's ability to understand language. Talk to him about nursing—especially if you are trying to postpone feedings. He may accept your wish to "save up the milk till nap time and night-night." Older toddlers may be able to agree to future weaning upon an upcoming birthday or other milestone, such as the start of preschool.

The bedtime nursing may continue as the child's favorite. Some mothers find this is a special time for themselves as well, and continue with it for weeks or months after other feedings have been abandoned. If you want to wean your toddler completely, your partner or another family member may be able to help the child establish a non-nursing bedtime routine.

Once nursings become infrequent, your breasts may look smaller and feel less firm. Still, you may be able to express milk for several months after nursing has stopped. Your breasts will probably regain their former size and shape within six months of weaning.

Whether you initiate weaning or whether it is a mutual undertaking, you are bound to feel a little sad as the final days of nursing arrive, marking the end of the precious time you and your child spent together nursing. I hope you will also feel proud of yourself, for the wonderful start in life that you have given your child.

Appendices

Appendix A: Resources for Nursing Mothers

Appendix B: Determining Babies' Milk
Needs during the First Six Weeks

Appendix C: The Safety of Drugs during
Breastfeeding

APPENDIX A

Resources for Nursing Mothers

Breastfeeding Support and Education

Nursing Mothers Counsel, Inc.
P.O. Box 50063
Palo Alto, California 94303
408-291-8008
www.nursingmothers.org

Nursing Mothers Counsel has chapters in various cities in northern
California. Call for a local number.

Boston Association for Childbirth Education (BACE)
Nursing Mothers' Council
P.O. Box 29
Newtonville, Massachusetts 02460
617-244-5102
www.bace-nmc.org

La Leche League International
1400 North Meacham Road
Schaumburg, Illinois 60173
800-LA LECHE
847-519-7730
www.lalecheleague.org

Call between 9:00 A.M. and 5:00 P.M. CST for breastfeeding help or a referral to a local La Leche League group. Most white pages list a local La Leche leader's phone number under "La Leche League."

Lactation Professional Referral Services

International Lactation Consultant Association
1500 Sunday Drive, Suite 102
Raleigh, North Carolina 27607
919-861-5577
www.ilca.org

Call weekdays between 9:00 A.M. and 5:00 P.M. EST, or, on the ILCA Web site, click on "Find an International Board-Certified Lactation Consultant in Your Area."

Breastfeeding National Network (Medela, Inc.)
800-TELL-YOU
www.medela.com

Call at any hour if you have Touch Tone dialing; if not, call weekdays between 7:30 A.M. and 6:00 P.M. CST.

International Board of Lactation Consultant Examiners
7309 Arlington Boulevard, Suite 300
Falls Church, Virginia 22042
703-560-7330
www.iblce.org

On the Web site, click on "U.S. regional registry."

Helpful Web Sites

www.babycenter.com
Thousands of original, medically reviewed articles on preconception, pregnancy, babies, and toddlers, plus live chats with experts, bulletin boards, and newsletters.

www.breastfeeding.com
Information, support, and resources for nursing mothers.

www.breastfeedingonline.com
Information for nursing mothers.

www.wiessinger.baka.com

Information for breastfeeding mothers and their helpers from Diane Wiessinger, a certified lactation consultant.

www.bfar.org

Information for women who are breastfeeding after breast reduction surgery.

www.fourfriends.com/abrw

Information for women who are or will be nursing adopted babies.

www.pumpingmoms.org

Discussion among breast-pump users, from occasional to full time. Topics include such matters as lactation problems and boosting the milk supply.

Special Supplemental Nutrition Program for Women, Infants, and Children (WIC)

WIC is a federally subsidized program that provides nutritional information, counseling, and food to low- and moderate-income pregnant and nursing mothers and their young children. Some WIC programs also offer breast pumps to nursing mothers. Eligibility for WIC is determined by family income, as shown in the chart. The income figures are adjusted yearly, so current figures may be higher if you are reading this after June 30, 2005. A pregnant woman may be counted as two in figuring eligibility.

WIC Income Requirements, May 1, 2004 to June 30, 2005

Number of persons in family	Maximum Gross Income			
	Annual	Monthly	Weekly	Hourly
1	$17,224	$1,436	$332	$ 8.28
2	23,107	1,926	445	11.11
3	28,990	2,416	558	13.94
4	34,873	2,907	671	16.77
5	40,756	3,397	784	19.59
6	46,639	3,887	897	22.42
7	52,522	4,377	1,011	25.25
8	58,405	4,868	1,124	28.08
over 8*	Add: 5,883	491	114	2.83

*For each additional family member, add the amount shown to the maximum gross income for a family of eight.

To locate a WIC office near your home, look for a listing in the phone book or contact your county or city health department.

Nursing Bras

Although nursing bras are available at maternity shops and department stores, the selection of styles and sizes may be too limited for you. The companies listed here sell nursing bras by mail- and phone-order. Call or write for their catalogs.

Motherwear
  320 Riverside Drive
  Northampton, Massachusetts 01062
  800-950-2500
  www.motherwear.com

Motherwear offers a wide variety of bra styles in sizes 32A to 48J.

Bosom Buddies, Inc.
  7332 South Alton Way, 13G
  Centennial, Colorado 80112
  720-482-0109
  888-860-0041
  www.bosombuddies.com

Bosom Buddies carries most brands of nursing bras, and will special-order from manufacturers as needed. The company provides fitting help by phone but is also willing to send bras in different sizes for you to try on; you can return those that don't fit.

Bravado! Designs
  41 Hollinger Road
  Toronto, Ontario M4B3G4
  Canada
  800-590-7802
  www.bravadodesigns.com

Bravado makes a comfortable, popular pull-on nursing bra of cotton and spandex, in five colors and in sizes from 32B to 46G. The company will custom-make larger sizes.

Medela
  P.O. Box 660
  McHenry, Illinois 60051
  800-435-8316
  www.medela.com

This leading breast-pump maker also carries soft-cup and underwire bras in sizes 32B to 46H, soft shoulder pads for use with any bra, and, for mothers who regularly pump their milk, a hands-free attachment kit for use with Medela bras. For referral to a local retailer, call 1-800-TELL-YOU.

Fancee Free Manufacturing Company
6609 Olive Boulevard
St. Louis, Missouri 63130
800-325-5088

Fancee Free carries many styles of nursing bras, in sizes 34C to 50K. Some styles have foam inserts for extra support and lift. Fancee Free bras are available in some maternity shops as well as by mail-order.

Electric Breast Pump Rental

Medela, Inc.
P.O. Box 660
McHenry, Illinois 60051
800-TELL-YOU
www.medela.com

Call at any hour if you have Touch Tone dialing; if not, call weekdays between 7:30 A.M. and 6:00 P.M. CST. Medela's Breastfeeding National Network will refer you to a local rental station where you can rent either a full-sized electric pump or the more portable Lactina Plus, a lightweight, fully automatic pump with an optional battery pack and an adapter for a car's cigarette lighter.

Hollister, Inc.
2000 Hollister Drive
Libertyville, Illinois 60048
800-323-4060
www.hollister.com

Call at any time to locate a pump rental station. Hollister will refer you to a local rental station where you can rent either a full-sized pump or the more portable Lact-E, a lightweight, fully automatic pump.

Breast Shells

Breast shells are used to correct inverted nipples during pregnancy and, sometimes, to protect injured nipples from friction against clothing. Many women find the flexible Soft Shells most effective and comfortable in treating inverted nipples. The Hobbit shells are vented to keep the nipples dry.

Medela Hobbit Breast Shells
Medela, Inc.
P.O. Box 660
McHenry, Illinois 60051
800-435-8316

$14.50 plus $4.00 shipping.

Medela Soft Shells
  Medela, Inc.
  P.O. Box 660
  McHenry, Illinois 60051
  800-435-8316
$17.50 per pair, plus $4.00 shipping.

Silicone Nursing Pads

An alternative to conventional cloth or disposable pads, these don't absorb milk but instead apply a gentle pressure on the nipple to keep milk from leaking. The pads adhere gently to the skin, so they can be worn without a bra.

LilyPadz
  Me & My Kidz
  P.O. Box 36
  Holland, Ohio 43528
  800-640-5454
  www.lilypadz.com
$19.95 plus $4.95 shipping. Call or visit the Web site to order or to locate a retailer near you.

Gel Dressings

These moist pads soothe sore and injured nipples and speed their healing.

Soothies
  990 Park Center Drive, Suite E
  Vista, California 92081
  800-922-4006
  E-mail: info@Soothies.com
$11.95 per pair. These glycerin gel pads are available at many drugstores. Call or e-mail to locate a local source.

Ameda ComfortGel Hydrogel Pads
  Hollister, Inc.
  2000 Hollister Drive
  Libertyville, Illinois 60048
  800-323-4060
$23 for a package of four. Call to order or to locate a retailer.

Breast Milk Coolers

These insulated coolers are used to store and transport breast milk.

Medela Cooler Carrier
  Medela, Inc.
  P.O. Box 660
  McHenry, Illinois 60051
  800-435-8316

$37.00 plus $7.00 shipping. This cooler has room for a small manual or battery-operated pump as well as an insulated area for milk.

Medela Lactina Cooler Carrier
  Medela, Inc.
  P.O. Box 660
  McHenry, Illinois 60051
  800-435-8316

$37.00 plus $4.00 shipping. This cooler has room for the Lactina pump as well as an insulated area for milk.

Nursing Supplementation Devices

A nursing supplementation device provides supplementary milk or formula while a baby is breastfeeding. Such a device is most commonly used when a baby is adopted or a mother wishes to relactate after a period of not nursing. It may also help when a mother wishes to both build up and supplement a low milk supply, or when a baby has a weak or ineffective suck.

A supplementer usually consists of a plastic pouch to hold breast milk or formula and a thin, flexible tube that is placed on the breast, ending at the nipple. The baby must latch on to the nipple and the soft tube. As the baby nurses, he receives the supplement along with whatever milk his mother is producing. These devices should be used with the guidance of a lactation professional experienced with them, and may also be available in your area through the same lactation professional. Medela and Lact-Aid will be happy to refer you to any local source. Currently they can also be ordered from:

Supplemental Nutrition System
  Medela, Inc.
  P.O. Box 660
  McHenry, Illinois 60051
  800-435-8316

$51.50 plus $4.00 shipping.

Lact-Aid International
P.O. Box 1066
Athens, Tennessee 37371
866-866-1239 (toll-free)
www.lact-aid.com

$42.00 plus shipping.

Domperidone (Motilium)

Usually sold for treating disorders of the gastrointestinal tract, this drug has also been found to stimulate milk production, more safely so than Reglan. Side effects in the mother (headache, abdominal cramps, dry mouth) are uncommon with domperidone, and very little of the medication reaches the baby.

With a prescription, domperidone can be made in the United States at special compounding pharmacies, but you can get it without a prescription and for a much lower cost from Global Health Ltd. in Vanuatu.

Global Health Ltd
877-271-6591 (toll-free)
011-678-28134
Fax: 011-678-28133
E-mail: admin@globalhealth.tv
www.globaldrug.tv

Order through the Web site or by fax, e-mail, or telephone. Prices are about 10 to 20 cents per 10-milligram tablet, depending on the quantity ordered (the minimum order is 100 tablets). Shipping to the United States takes 10 to 14 days.

Nursing Pillows

My Brest Friend Nursing Pillow
35 Leveroni Court
Novato, California 94949
415-883-5300
www.mybrestfriend.com

$39.95. This wearable pillow with a cushioned back support makes positioning the baby easier and sitting to nurse more comfortable. Call or check the Web site to find a dealer near you.

Nurse EZ Plus Twin Pillow
  Basic Comfort, Inc.
  4100 Grape Street, Unit 2
  Denver, Colorado 80216
  800-456-8687
$35.00 plus $7.30 shipping.

Nursing Stool

Medela Nursing Stool
  Medela, Inc.
  P.O. Box 660
  McHenry, Illinois 60051
  800-435-8316
$30.00 plus $10.00 shipping.

Modified Lanolin

Lansinoh
  Lansinoh Laboratories
  333 North Fairfax St., Suite 400
  Alexandria, Virginia 22314
  888-607-4287

$9.99 for a 2-ounce tube, plus shipping and handling. Call to order or to locate a local source. Lansinoh is carried at many drugstores and discount stores.

Pur-Lan 100
  Medela, Inc.
  P.O. Box 660
  McHenry, Illinois 60051
  800-435-8316
$2.50 for ¼ ounce; $7.00 for 1.3 ounces. Include $4.00 for shipping.

Electronic Baby Scale

Medela, Inc.
  P.O. Box 660
  McHenry, Illinois 60051
  800-435-8316

Ask for the name of a nearby rental station or order directly from the company. Renting a scale costs approximately $35.00 per week.

Haberman Feeder

This feeder is designed for babies with cleft palates or other problems that make feeding difficult. Minimal effort is required for the baby to obtain milk.

Medela, Inc.
   P.O. Box 660
   McHenry, Illinois 60051
   800-435-8316
$25.50 plus $4.00 shipping.

Breast Milk Storage Bags

These bags are constructed for leak-free milk storage. They are sturdier than bottle liners, which are often used for milk storage. To save time, milk bags can be used in place of bottles while pumping.

Mother's Milk Storage Bags
   Breastfeeding Support Network
   2050 West Ninth Avenue
   Oshkosh, Wisconsin 54904
   888-666-7224
For 25 bags, $8.95 plus $2.00 shipping.

Mother's Milk Freezer Bags
   Hollister, Inc.
   2000 Hollister Drive
   Libertyville, Illinois 60048
   800-323-4060
   www.ameda.com
For 20 bags, $11.50. Call or check the Web site to find a local retailer.

Attachable Baby Bed

The Arm's Reach Bedside Co-Sleeper is a baby bed that connects to a full-size bed to allow a mother and her baby to sleep safely and comfortably next to each other. For beds higher than 24 inches from the floor, a leg extension kit is available separately.

Arm's Reach Concepts
2081 North Oxnard Boulevard, PMB #187
Oxnard, California 93030
800-954-9353
www.armsreach.com

Various models are available. Priced from $146 to $299, they can be converted into a bassinet, a playpen, a changing table, or even a love seat. Visit the Arm's Reach Web site to find a local retailer.

Milk Banks

While some women are unable to produce sufficient milk, others produce more than their babies can use. Therein lies the beauty of a milk bank, which serves both those in need of milk and those who wish to donate it.

Women who wish to donate milk must be healthy nonsmokers who take no medications (with some exceptions). Most milk banks require a minimum number of ounces from each donor.

Donors freeze their milk before taking it to the milk bank. There the milk is thawed, pooled with that of other donors, heat-treated to kill any bacteria or viruses, and re-frozen (it retains its immunological properties through this processing). The milk is dispensed only after a cultured sample shows no bacterial growth. Then is it shipped frozen by overnight express to hospitals and individual recipients.

Because of all the work that goes into processing it, donated milk is expensive, and its supply is limited. Parents who want to buy donated milk must have a physician's prescription. Common conditions for which physicians prescribe donated milk include prematurity, allergies, formula intolerance, immunological deficiencies, infectious diseases, and inborn errors of metabolism. Doctors may also prescribe donated milk for short periods to provide superior nutrition for a baby recovering from surgery or to get an adopted baby off to a good start.

There are currently six milk banks in the United States and one in Canada:

CALIFORNIA
Mothers' Milk Bank at Valley
Medical Center
  751 South Bascom Avenue
  San Jose, California 95128
  408-998-4550
  Fax: 408-297-9208

COLORADO
Mothers' Milk Bank at Presbyterian
St. Luke's Medical Center
  1719 East 19th Avenue
  Denver, Colorado 80218
  303-869-1888
  Fax: 303-869-2490

DELAWARE
Mothers' Milk Bank
Christiana Care Health System
  Christiana Hospital
  4755 Ogletown-Stanton Road
  Newark, Delaware 19718
  302-733-2340
  Fax: 302-733-2396

IOWA
Mothers' Milk Bank of Iowa
  Division of Nutrition
  Department of Pediatrics
  Children's Hospital of Iowa
  200 Hawkins Drive
  Iowa City, Iowa 52242
  877-891-5347 (toll free)
  Fax: 319-353-7598

NORTH CAROLINA
Mothers' Milk Bank at WakeMed
  3000 New Bern Avenue
  Raleigh, North Carolina 27610
  919-350-8599
  Fax: 919-350-8923

TEXAS
Mothers' Milk Bank at Austin
  900 East 30th Street, Suite 214
  Austin, Texas 78705
  512-494-0800
  Fax: 512-494-0880

BRITISH COLUMBIA
BC Women's Milk Bank
  C&W Lactation Services
  4450 Oak Street, IU 30
  Vancouver, British Columbia
  V6M 3X4
  604-875-2282
  Fax: 604-875-2871

APPENDIX B

DETERMINING BABIES' MILK NEEDS DURING THE FIRST SIX WEEKS

Ten Percent Weight Loss

A newborn should lose less than 10 percent of her birth weight before she begins to gain weight. Find your baby's birth weight in the left column of the table. Look at the figure across from your baby's birth weight in the right column. If your baby weighs this amount or less, you'll want to compare her milk needs (see the following sections of this appendix) with your milk production, and take steps to increase her milk intake.

Birth Weight (in pounds-ounces)	10% Less	Birth Weight (in pounds-ounces)	10% Less	Birth Weight (in pounds-ounces)	10% Less
4-8	4-2	7-0	6-5	9-8	8-9
4-9	4-2.5	7-1	6-6	9-9	8-10
4-10	4-3	7-2	6-7	9-10	8-10.5
4-11	4-3.5	7-3	6-7.5	9-11	8-11.5
4-12	4-4	7-4	6-8	9-12	8-12
4-13	4-5	7-5	6-9	9-13	8-13
4-14	4-6	7-6	6-10	9-14	8-14
4-15	4-7	7-7	6-11	9-15	8-15
5-0	4-8	7-8	6-12	10-0	9-0
5-1	4-9	7-9	6-13	10-1	9-1
5-2	4-10	7-10	6-14	10-2	9-2
5-3	4-11	7-11	6-15	10-3	9-3
5-4	4-12	7-12	7-0	10-4	9-4
5-5	4-12.5	7-13	7-0.5	10-5	9-4.5
5-6	4-13	7-14	7-1	10-6	9-5
5-7	4-14	7-15	7-2	10-7	9-6
5-8	4-15	8-0	7-3	10-8	9-7
5-9	5-0	8-1	7-4	10-9	9-8
5-10	5-1	8-2	7-5	10-10	9-9
5-11	5-2	8-3	7-6	10-11	9-10
5-12	5-3	8-4	7-7	10-12	9-11
5-13	5-4	8-5	7-8	10-13	9-12
5-14	5-5	8-6	7-9	10-14	9-13
5-15	5-5.5	8-7	7-9.5	10-15	9-13.5
6-0	5-6	8-8	7-10	11-0	9-14.5
6-1	5-7	8-9	7-11	11-1	9-15
6-2	5-8	8-10	7-12	11-2	10-0
6-3	5-9	8-11	7-13	11-3	10-1
6-4	5-10	8-12	7-14	11-4	10-2
6-5	5-11	8-13	7-15	11-5	10-3
6-6	5-12	8-14	8-0	11-6	10-4
6-7	5-13	8-15	8-1	11-7	10-5
6-8	5-14	9-0	8-2	11-8	10-5.5
6-9	5-14.5	9-1	8-2.5	11-9	10-6.5
6-10	5-15	9-2	8-3	11-10	10-7.5
6-11	6-0	9-3	8-4	11-11	10-8
6-12	6-1	9-4	8-5	11-12	10-9
6-13	6-2	9-5	8-6	11-13	10-10
6-14	6-3	9-6	8-7	11-14	10-11
6-15	6-4	9-7	8-8	11-15	10-12

Babies' Milk Needs during the First Five Days

Find your baby's age in the left column. At right is the amount of milk he needs at each of eight daily feedings.

	Milk Needed per Feeding	
Baby's Age, in Hours	*in Milliliters*	*in Ounces*
24–48	15	1/2
48–72	20	2/3
72–96	30	1
96–120	45	1 1/2

Babies' Milk Needs from Five Days to Six Weeks of Age

Follow these steps to determine how much milk your baby needs.

Step 1. Weigh the baby naked, on an accurate scale, at least one hour after a feeding. Find the baby's weight in kilograms in the chart below. If the baby weighs 7 pounds, 5 ounces, for example, look down the column headed "7" and across the row headed "5." The baby's weight in kilograms is 3.317.

	Pounds										
Ounces	4	5	6	7	8	9	10	11	12	13	14
0	1.814	2.268	2.722	3.175	3.629	4.082	4.536	4.990	5.443	5.897	6.350
1	1.843	2.296	2.750	3.203	3.657	4.111	4.564	5.018	5.471	5.925	6.379
2	1.871	2.325	2.778	3.232	3.685	4.139	4.593	5.046	5.500	5.953	6.407
3	1.899	2.353	2.807	3.260	3.714	4.167	4.621	5.075	5.528	5.982	6.435
4	1.928	2.381	2.835	3.289	3.742	4.196	4.649	5.103	5.557	6.010	6.464
5	1.956	2.410	2.863	3.317	3.770	4.224	4.678	5.131	5.585	6.038	6.492
6	1.984	2.438	2.892	3.345	3.799	4.252	4.706	5.160	5.613	6.067	6.520
7	2.013	2.466	2.920	3.374	3.827	4.281	4.734	5.188	5.642	6.095	6.549
8	2.041	2.495	2.948	3.402	3.856	4.309	4.763	5.216	5.670	6.123	6.577
9	2.070	2.523	2.977	3.430	3.884	4.337	4.791	5.245	5.698	6.152	6.605
10	2.098	2.551	3.005	3.459	3.912	4.366	4.819	5.273	5.727	6.180	6.634
11	2.126	2.580	3.033	3.487	3.941	4.394	4.848	5.301	5.755	6.209	6.662
12	2.155	2.608	3.062	3.515	3.969	4.423	4.876	5.330	5.783	6.237	6.690
13	2.183	2.637	3.090	3.544	3.997	4.451	4.904	5.358	5.812	6.265	6.719
14	2.211	2.665	3.118	3.572	4.026	4.479	4.933	5.386	5.840	6.294	6.747
15	2.240	2.693	3.147	3.600	4.054	4.508	4.961	5.415	5.868	6.322	6.776

Step 2. To determine the approximate amount of milk a baby needs in a 24-hour period, multiply the baby's weight in kilograms by 6, and round the result to the nearest whole number.

Example: 3.317 kilograms x 6 = 19.902 ounces

If the baby weighs 3.317 kilograms, she needs approximately 20 ounces of milk per day.

Step 3. Calculate how much milk the baby needs at each feeding. Divide the amount of milk the baby needs daily by the number of times she nurses in each 24-hour period.

Example: 20 ounces ÷ 8 = 2$\frac{1}{2}$ ounces

If the baby needs 20 ounces of milk per day and nurses eight times per day, she needs 2$\frac{1}{2}$ ounces of milk at each feeding.

If the baby is taking eight feedings per day, however, you can skip step two, and instead multiply the baby's current weight in kilograms by 22.5. The result will be the amount of milk the baby needs at each feeding in milliliters.

Example: 3.317 kilograms x 22.5 = 74.6325 milliliters

A baby weighing 3.317 kilograms needs approximately 75 milliliters of milk per feeding. To find this amount in ounces, divide by 30.

Example: 75 milliliters ÷ 30 = 2$\frac{1}{2}$ ounces

The baby in our example needs 2$\frac{1}{2}$ ounces of milk at each of eight daily feedings.

If the baby is taking nine feedings every 24 hours, you can find how much milk she needs at each feeding by multiplying her weight in kilograms by 20.

Example: 3.317 kilograms x 20 = 66.34 milliliters

The baby weighing 3.317 kilograms and nursing nine times per day needs about 66 milliliters of milk at each feeding.

Example: 66 milliliters ÷ 30 = 2.2 ounces

Since 30 milliliters equals 1 ounce, the baby needs 2$\frac{1}{5}$ ounces of milk nine times per day.

APPENDIX C

THE SAFETY OF DRUGS DURING BREASTFEEDING

By Philip O. Anderson, Pharm.D., F.A.S.H.P., F.C.S.H.P.

If you are considering taking a drug while nursing, you are likely wondering what effects it may have on your baby and on milk production. Clear guidelines are sometimes hard to come by in this situation. This appendix will explain what you should consider before taking a particular drug, and how, if you take it, you can minimize its effects on your child.

The passage of drugs into milk   Almost any drug you take will reach your milk in some quantity. Although you would never want to expose your baby to a foreign chemical unnecessarily, the amount of a drug that appears in milk is usually not great enough to harm a nursing child. One group of researchers found that 87 percent of drugs are transmitted in amounts of 10 percent or less of the mother's dose. Only about 3 percent of drugs reach the infant in amounts similar to the mother's dose.

Several considerations are important when deciding whether to take a particular drug.

Your baby's age and maturity. Just as your baby becomes better able to move about as he grows older, his ability to metabolize and detoxify foreign chemicals and drugs improves with time. Premature infants have little ability to metabolize drugs; when a premie needs treatment for a medical condition, drugs are given in much smaller doses than they would be for a full-term newborn or an older infant. The amount of medication in a mother's milk that is safe for a one-month-old might be dangerous for a premature infant. Likewise, a baby who is several months old has a much greater capability of handling drugs in breast milk than does a one-month-old. And when an infant begins to eat solid food he consumes less breast milk and, therefore, less of any drug it may contain. Most unwanted drug reactions in breastfed infants occur when the babies are less than two months old—most often in the first month. It is rare for medications in breast milk to affect infants over six months old.

Your needs. Maybe you have a serious medical condition that threatens your health and your ability to care for your child, and you must take medication for it. Or maybe you're suffering from only a minor discomfort, and can get by without a medication. Whatever your condition, you must evaluate its seriousness and the consequences of not taking a particular drug. Then weigh these consequences against the benefits of breastfeeding, as you see them. You may decide to pump your milk and discard it while you're taking the medication or, if necessary, give up nursing altogether rather than expose your baby to a potentially hazardous drug. Only infrequently does a mother's medication make it necessary for a mother to completely stop nursing, though. Researchers in Canada found that many mothers who were prescribed an antibiotic for an infection failed to take the medication for fear of harming their nursing infants, even after being told that the drug was safe to use during nursing. Such action could easily cause a resurgence of the infection and the need for a more potent antibiotic.

The duration of treatment. If you have a chronic health problem, such as high blood pressure, you may be taking a drug over a long period. But perhaps you need medication for only a few days, as is usual with many antibiotics, or even just once, as with an anesthetic for a dental procedure or a diagnostic agent for an X-ray. If only brief drug therapy is needed, you can usually avoid exposing your infant to harmful amounts of the drug with minimal disruption to your normal pattern of breastfeeding.

The history of the drug. If a drug has been used for many years—especially if it has been given frequently to infants or to nursing mothers—the risks it poses to the breastfed baby are quite predictable. This is not so, however, for drugs that are new on the market, most herbal remedies, and for drugs that have never been used in children or infants. With no safety record to go on, health-care providers may vary in their assessments of the risks your baby faces from small amounts of the drug in your milk. Drugs given to you as samples by your physician are usually very new and are unlikely to have information about use during breastfeeding. Ask your physician if she can prescribe an older medication that will be just as effective as the sample of the new drug—the peace of mind is usually worth the cost of paying for the prescription.

You may also get different advice from different physicians—your obstetrician and the baby's pediatrician, for example. Unnecessary alarm and confusion is often caused by statements concerning nursing made by a drug's manufacturer in the *Physician's Desk Reference (PDR)* or package insert. These statements generally are not written to help the nursing mother; instead, they usually reflect the manufacturer's desire for protection from legal liability. Unfortunately, many health-care providers use the *PDR* as their primary source of information on the use of drugs during lactation. Many mothers stop nursing after receiving such confusing or inaccurate advice. It is important to consult a health professional with expertise in advising nursing mothers about medication use if you have questions about your drug.

The persistence of the drug in the body. Some drugs are eliminated from the body after only a few hours, whereas others remain a long time and accumulate. Accumulation potential is measured by the "half-life" of the drug; it takes four to five half-lives for a drug to be eliminated from the body. Drugs with long half-lives are more likely to persist in milk than are those with short half-lives. Long-acting drugs are also more likely to accumulate in the baby and affect her health.

Coordinating feedings and dosage. If a drug is short-acting, or quickly eliminated, you may be able to time the doses in a way that will minimize the amount of drug in your milk at feedings. You might take a dose just after nursing, so the amount of drug in the milk peaks between feedings. If you are on a once-a-day medication, you might take it after the last feeding of the evening, and substitute milk expressed during the day for the nighttime feedings; by morning the amount of drug in your milk may be down to an acceptably low level. These strategies work best with older infants who are nursing at infrequent intervals.

Part of the reason you can limit your baby's drug exposure this way is that drugs pass in both directions between your bloodstream and breast milk. As the drug levels in your bloodstream decrease, the drug in your milk will pass back into your bloodstream. When breastfeeding must be withheld because of drug therapy that may harm an infant, expressing and discarding milk ("pumping and dumping") is sometimes advocated in the mistaken belief that the drug will thereby be eliminated from the milk sooner. Because of the reverse passage of drugs from milk to the bloodstream and because only a very small fraction of the drug in your body is in your milk, pumping and dumping has very little effect on the eventual amount of drug your baby gets from your milk. Pumping the breasts may be useful, though, in maintaining your milk supply and decreasing any pain from engorgement when you've temporarily stopped breastfeeding.

Route of administration. The way that you take a medication partially determines how much of the drug will get into your bloodstream and to your baby. Drugs you're given by injection go directly into your bloodstream and can reach the milk, but some injected drugs cannot be absorbed into the infant's bloodstream from her gastrointestinal tract. Medications you take by mouth usually appear in your bloodstream, except for some that are meant to work locally in the stomach or intestines. Significant amounts of drugs can be absorbed from drops and ointments placed in the eye. Vaginal and rectal products can also be absorbed into the bloodstream. Drugs taken by inhaler generally reach the bloodstream in smaller amounts than the same drug taken orally.

Since creams and ointments applied to the skin usually do not allow very much drug into your bloodstream, they are generally safe to use while nursing. Be careful, though, not to get a medicated cream on your baby's skin or allow him to get any into his mouth. If you are applying medication to your nipples, wet the area with a small amount of expressed breast milk and wipe gently before nursing to remove any residual medication. You can reapply the medication after nursing. It is better to use water-washable creams on the breast than petrolatum (Vaseline)-based ointments, because the baby can ingest and absorb some of the petroleum-based oils found in petrolatum.

The effects of drugs on lactation

Not only may the drugs you take affect your baby directly, but some may influence your milk production. This can happen in a number of ways, since several hormones work together to control lactation. Some drugs are used deliberately to stimulate or stop milk flow; however, a few medications intended for another purpose have been shown to affect lactation. Those that have are identified in this appendix.

Side effects in the baby

Only infrequently must nursing be discontinued completely because of potential drug toxicity. Concern usually arises when the baby is a newborn or when the mother must take one of the most toxic drugs. But even drugs that are usually safe for nursing babies can occasionally cause mild but unpredictable allergic reactions, such as skin rashes. Minor side effects such as fussiness, drowsiness, and diarrhea occur sometimes, but usually do not require medical attention. More serious side effects are rare.

If side effects or possible allergies become a problem for your baby while you're taking a drug, do not hesitate to seek help.

Common drugs and their safety

In the following list, common drugs are grouped into categories and subcategories according to their uses. Noted are their potential effects on the breastfeeding infant and, where applicable, on lactation itself. Drug names that begin with a lower-case letter are generic; those that begin with a capital letter are brand names. A more complete listing of brand names is in the "Index to Common Drugs" on page 280. If you can't find the drug you're looking for here or need more specific information, you might call the University of California San Diego Drug Information Service at 619-543-6971. Hours for this service are Monday through Friday, 9:00 A.M. to 5:00 P.M. PST.

Acne products. Even though the manufacturer warns against it, *tretinoin* is safe to use during nursing if it is applied only to the face. Avoid touching the infant's skin with treated areas of your own skin, when you're nursing and when you're not. Other topical products, such as *benzoyl peroxide, clindamycin,* and *erythromycin* are also safe. *Isotretinoin,* which is taken by mouth, should not be used while nursing. Daily long-term use (more than two weeks) of *tetracycline* for acne is not desirable while nursing.

Anesthetics

General anesthetics. Nitrous oxide is sometimes used for dental procedures and short outpatient procedures; it is rapidly eliminated from the milk. Injectable anesthetics such as *midazolam, propofol,* and *thiopental,* which are used for many short, outpatient surgical procedures, have little or no effect on breastfed infants. Gaseous general anesthetics such as *desflurane, enflurane, halothane, isoflurane,* and *sevoflurane,* which are used in hospitals for major operations, have not been studied in nursing mothers and their babies. These drugs persist in the body longer than nitrous oxide, but appear unlikely to affect breastfed infants because they have to be inhaled in relatively large amounts to work—your baby will get only small amounts by mouth. Generally, by the time a mother feels sufficiently recovered from anesthesia to breastfeed, it is safe to resume nursing.

Local anesthetics. These drugs are given by injection for dental or other short procedures. Although many people refer to all of these drugs as "Novocaine" (the trade name for *procaine*), this old drug is rarely used now. Information on the effects of local anesthetics during nursing is available for only two drugs, *lidocaine* and *bupivacaine,* both of which are safe to use while nursing. Ask your physician or dentist if one of these can be used. Although other local anesthetics are unlikely to affect a breastfed baby, breastfeeding may be withheld as a precaution for four hours after one of these other drugs is administered.

Antibacterials. Most drugs that are taken for infections reach the milk in only small quantities—quantities that would be too small to treat the same infections in your infant. Occasionally, though, these small drug amounts can disrupt the normal balance of microorganisms in a baby's mouth and intestines. This may result in diarrhea or diaper rash, caused by an overgrowth of yeast or other organisms in the bowel or, less often, thrush, an overgrowth of yeast in the mouth (see "Thrush Nipples," page 53, and "Fussiness, Colic, and Reflux," page 152). Although these conditions generally are not serious and can be readily treated, it is important to watch for their signs while you are taking an antibacterial drug, especially if you need more than one course of therapy for a persistent infection.

The likelihood of diarrhea or thrush occurring depends on the particular drug you are taking. Some antibacterials may also cause other problems. In the unlikely event that blood appears in your infant's stool, stop breastfeeding, and call your physician immediately.

Aminoglycosides. These drugs (*gentamicin, tobramycin, amikacin*) are given primarily in the hospital, by injection. Amounts that appear in milk are very small and pose no special risk to the breastfed infant.

Cephalosporins. These are similar to penicillins, and the same precautions apply. Occasionally allergies develop, so watch for signs of rash. Cephalosporins, especially the more potent ones given by injection, may cause diarrhea and thrush. *Cephalexin* and *cefuroxime* are commonly prescribed cephalosporins.

Clindamycin. Clindamycin is best avoided if possible, but a few days of therapy is probably safe, as long as the baby is closely monitored for diarrhea and bloody stools. Clindamycin presents less risk to the infant if it is given vaginally rather than orally or intravenously. See also "Acne Products," page 257.

Erythromycins. Erythromycin is a generally safe drug that is often given directly to infants. The closely related drugs *azithromycin* and *clarithromycin* appear to be equally safe. Watch for signs of jaundice (yellowing of the skin and eyes) and contact your physician if this occurs. See also "Acne Products," page 257.

Furazolidone. This drug is poorly absorbed into the bloodstream after oral use. It is a good alternative to metronidazole for *Giardia* infections if your infant is more than one month old.

Isoniazid. This drug, used to treat tuberculosis, enters the milk in small amounts. It poses a slight risk of damage to the baby's liver. Treating the mother with the drug, however, is safer than exposing the infant to tuberculosis. Watch the infant for signs of jaundice (yellowing of the skin and eyes) and contact your physician if this occurs.

Metronidazole. Breastfeeding should be stopped temporarily during use of this medication, but can be resumed 24 hours after the last dose. In the treatment of *Trichomonas* infections, metronidazole can be given as a single dose. For *Giardia* infections, a better alternative is furazolidone if the infant is over one month old. For postoperative (including C-section) infections, consider *clindamycin* as an alternative.

Nitrofurantoin. This drug appears in small amounts in breast milk; these amounts are generally not harmful to infants over one month of age, but the drug should be avoided with younger babies.

Penicillins. These are very safe drugs that are often given directly to infants as treatment for infections. Occasionally allergies develop to penicillins, so the baby should be watched for rashes. If you see signs of rash, diarrhea, or thrush, call your health-care provider. If your infant has previously had a rash or other reaction to a penicillin, you should not take a penicillin while breastfeeding.

Quinolones. Ciprofloxacin, levofloxacin, gatifloxacin, moxifloxacin (and several others) have not been well studied in nursing infants because they are usually not given directly to infants or children. Recent experience in infants and children indicates that they are probably not particularly harmful during nursing. *Norfloxacin* is a quinolone that is excreted into milk in lesser amounts than others and is poorly absorbed by the infant. Norfloxacin is sometimes a good alternative for urinary tract infections during nursing.

Sulfonamides (sulfas). Septra and *Bactrim* are common drugs that contain *trimethorprim* and the sulfonamide *sulfamethoxazole. Sulfisoxazole* is another common sulfa. Large doses of sulfas given directly to newborn infants can increase the risk of jaundice (yellowing of the skin and eyes). Other medications are usually preferred if the baby is premature or under two months of age. Combination tablets containing the red dye *phenazopyridine*, such as *Azo-Gantrisin* or *Azo-Gantanol*, should be avoided, particularly with newborns. Phenazopyridine is also the ingredient in *Pyridium*. This drug decreases pain on urination, but is not necessary to treat a bladder infection.

Tetracyclines. These are generally not given to children or pregnant women because they can cause permanent staining of the infant's teeth. The amounts that appear in milk, however, are very small and are somewhat inactivated by the calcium in milk. In fact, tooth staining caused by a tetracycline in breast milk has never been reported. Tetracyclines can be used safely by the nursing mother for short periods (two weeks or less), but should be used only if no other drug will work. One tetracycline, *minocycline*, can cause the milk to turn black. See also "Acne Products," page 257.

Vancomycin. This drug is excreted into milk in only small amounts and is not absorbed into the baby's bloodstream. Vancomycin is safe during nursing.

Anticoagulants. Some anticoagulants (such as *heparin, enoxaparin,* and *dalteparin*) are injected; others (such as *warfarin*) are taken orally. Injected anticoagulants can be safely used during lactation because they do not pass well into milk nor get well absorbed by the nursing infant. Although warfarin was thought for many years to endanger the breastfeeding infant, newer evidence indicates that this oral drug is acceptable as well; only small amounts are found in breast milk.

Ticlopidine and *clopidogrel* act in a different way to decrease blood platelet function. Neither has been studied during nursing, and so they both should be avoided.

Anticonvulsants. Anticonvulsants are used to treat epilepsy, mood disorders, and nerve pain. Because these medications are used continuously and are often long-acting, they should be taken with caution during breastfeeding. Your baby may show no effects other than subtle behavioral changes, so be vigilant. Infants of mothers taking anticonvulsants tend to have more difficulty nursing and tend to wean earlier than average. You may need to have your infant's blood drawn to determine if the drug is affecting her.

Carbamazepine. This drug is known to pass into milk in significant amounts. Although breastfed infants of women taking the drug usually show no effects from it, two such infants have had liver problems. Watch for jaundice (yellowing of the skin and eyes) while using carbamazepine.

Clonazepam. There is not much information on the effects of this benzodiazepine drug during breastfeeding, but it may make the baby drowsy.

Gabapentin. There is no information available about the appearance of gabapentin in breast milk.

Lamotrigine. Breastfed infants of women taking lamotrigine have relatively high blood levels of this drug. One breastfed newborn infant became very drowsy when his mother began taking it. Lamotrigine also can cause very severe skin reactions, so use it with caution until more information is available.

Levetiracetam. Only one breastfeeding mother who took this drug has been studied, and she excreted rather large amounts in milk. This drug should be used with caution during lactation.

Oxcarbazepine. Only one infant has been reported to have been breastfed while the mother used oxcarbazepine. The infant did well during four months of nursing. Use this drug with caution until more information is available.

Phenobarbital. This drug has been given directly to infants for many years, usually with no severe adverse effects. You can probably use it safely during breastfeeding, although it may make the baby drowsy and less interested in nursing. The baby's behavior, weight gain, and blood levels should be monitored if there is concern. Women taking phenobarbital sometimes have to stop nursing because of its effects on their infants.

Phenytoin. This drug has been used for many years by breastfeeding women. It is usually safe, because very low amounts pass into breast milk.

Primidone. This drug is similar to phenobarbital; the same precautions apply.

Topiramate. Two infants have been breastfed by women who took this drug, and no adverse effects have been reported. Use topiramate with caution until more information is available.

Valproic acid. Only very small amounts of this drug enter milk; rarely, however, the drug may cause liver damage or interference with blood platelets. Infants should be watched for unusual bruising or signs of jaundice (yellowing of the skin and eyes).

Zonisamide. Information comes from only three mother-infant pairs. Use caution with this drug until more information is available.

Antifungals

Clotrimazole (dissolved from a troche) and *miconazole* have been safely used in the mouths of infants with thrush, often successfully after nystatin has failed, and these antifungals are also safe to use for vaginal infections. Numerous related drugs, such as *butoconazole, terconazole,* and *tioconazole* are also available for vaginal use. Since little is known about their absorption into the bloodstream of a nursing infant, it is preferable to use clotrimazole or miconazole when a vaginal antifungal is needed.

Fluconazole. Fluconazole is a potent, low-risk antifungal that is taken orally. A single dose for vaginal infections is safe while nursing. This drug can also be used simultaneously in the mother and infant to treat breast infections and thrush when other drugs have failed. At least two weeks of therapy is required in this situation.

Ketoconazole. You should not take ketoconazole orally or apply it to your nipples, because it can be absorbed into the baby's bloodstream and may be toxic.

Polyenes. Since *Amphotericin B* and *nystatin* aren't absorbed into the baby's bloodstream, you can safely use them in your infant's mouth or on your nipples to treat thrush (*Candida* infections), or you can take them by mouth yourself.

Antinauseants. Most drugs used for nausea and vomiting are pheno-thiazine derivatives (see "Psychotherapeutic Agents," page 275), such as *prochlorperazine, promethazine,* and *thiethylperazine,* taken in low doses. Another commonly used drug is *trimethobenzamide.* These drugs may cause transient drowsiness or, rarely, abnormal movements in infants, but are safe to use for a short time. Newer antinauseants such as *dolasetron, ondansetron,* and *granisetron* are used for more severe nausea due to cancer chemotherapy or general anesthesia. Although these drugs have not been studied in breastfeeding women, we know that if they do get into the mother's milk they will not be absorbed well into the baby's bloodstream. The risk they pose to the baby, therefore, seems minimal.

Antiparasitics. Insecticides are used to treat scabies, a skin condition caused by mites, and pediculosis, or infestation with lice. An old medica-tion, *lindane,* is a very fat-soluble insecticide that can persist in milk and in the baby's body a long time. Although no harm has been reported in breastfed infants due to lindane, this drug is best avoided. Safer alternatives include *pyrethrins (Rid* and *A-200,* for example) or *permethrin (Nix)* for lice, and a higher potency permethrin (*Elimite*) for scabies.

Mebendazole. Mebendazole is used for various worm (parasite) infestations. Since it is poorly absorbed from the intestinal tract, it is unlikely to cause adverse effects in breastfed infants. Contrary to an old report, it does not inhibit lactation.

Antivirals

Acyclovir. This antiviral drug is sometimes used to treat newborns. When taken by a breastfeeding mother, it is well tolerated by the baby.

Amantadine. This antiviral agent for influenza should be avoided during nursing, since it may decrease milk production and cause side effects in the breastfed baby.

Famciclovir. Famciclovir and its derivative, *penciclovir* (which is available as a topical cream), have not been studied in infants or during nursing. Acyclovir or valaciclovir is a safer alternative for a herpes infection.

Valaciclovir. Valaciclovir breaks down in the mother's body to acyclovir, so the information on acyclovir also applies to valaciclovir. It is safe to use during nursing.

Arthritis, pain, and migraine medications

Acetaminophen. This drug is often used in infants and is safe to use during breastfeeding.

Antirheumatic drugs. Etanercept, infliximab, and *leflunomide* are used for severe rheumatoid arthritis. These drugs have not been studied well during breastfeeding and are potentially harmful to the baby's immune system and organs. At this time, therefore, these drugs are usually considered incompatible with breastfeeding. Some very preliminary information indicates that etanercept might be compatible with nursing.

Aspirin. When large doses are taken daily, as for arthritis, problems can sometimes occur. Generally, it is best to avoid aspirin; ibuprofen is a better choice. If you take an occasional aspirin, do not breastfeed for at least one hour after the dose.

Ergotamine. This is a component of several products, such as *Cafergot,* used in the treatment of migraine headaches. Some ergot alkaloids cause vomiting in breastfed infants whose mothers have taken the drugs. Although ergotamine itself has not been studied, avoiding it while breastfeeding seems prudent (see "Triptans," page 264).

Narcotics. Drowsiness due to narcotics in milk occurs more commonly in infants than formerly thought: About 20 percent of breastfed babies whose mothers have taken narcotics are affected. The degree of drowsiness varies with the dosage, and babies less than one month old are particularly susceptible. Limiting the dosage to one tablet (such as 30 milligrams of *codeine*, 5 milligrams of *hydrocodone* or *oxycodone*, or 65 milligrams of *propoxyphene*) every four hours is advisable; acetaminophen or ibuprofen can be taken in addition. Single injections of narcotics during nursing usually cause no problems, but intravenous narcotics given during labor can sometimes interfere with the establishment of lactation. *Meperidine* is the worst in this regard; *morphine* causes fewer problems, and *fentanyl* the least. Epidural administration causes fewer problems in nursing infants. *Tramadol* has not been well studied, but apparently only a small amount appears in milk. *Methadone*, when used for maintenance in narcotic addicts, appears not to harm their breastfed infants. When a mother has taken methadone during pregnancy, the methadone in her breast milk minimizes the methadone withdrawal symptoms in her newborn.

Nonsteroidal anti-inflammatory drugs (NSAIDs). Ibuprofen, diclofenac, and *flurbiprofen* appear in only minute amounts in milk; they seem safe to use while nursing an infant of any age. If your infant is more than one month old, you can also safely use *fenoprofen, ketoprofen, naproxen, tolmetin*, and long-acting drugs such as *diflunisal, piroxicam*, and *sulindac*. The more toxic drugs *ketorolac, mefenamic acid*, and *indomethacin* should be avoided during breastfeeding. Of the newer COX-II inhibitors (*celecoxib, rofecoxib, valdecoxib*), only celecoxib has been studied, and only in one mother-infant pair. Levels in milk are low, and these drugs are less toxic than the older NSAIDs, so it is unlikely that these drugs pose a risk to the nursing infant. Until more information becomes available, however, ibuprofen is the best choice among the NSAIDs.

"Triptans." Very little *sumatriptan* appears in milk, even when it is given by injection, and the small amount that reaches the infant is poorly absorbed. Similar drugs for migraine (*naratriptan, rizatriptan*, and *zolmitriptan*) have not been studied, so sumatriptan is preferable to these.

Bisphosphonates. These drugs are used to treat and prevent osteoporosis and to decrease bone loss during cancer chemotherapy. Drugs in this class include *alendronate, etidronate, pamidronate, risedronate, tiludronate*, and *zoledronic acid*. Since only very small amounts of pamidronate are excreted into breast milk, it is a preferred drug. Because zoledronic acid binds to bones for an extremely long time, it should not be used during breastfeeding.

Cancer chemotherapy. This group includes the drugs used to treat cancer, severe arthritis, and certain skin diseases. Because these agents are among the most toxic used in medicine, very few women have breastfed while taking them. Little is known about the passage of these drugs into milk, but even small amounts, should they reach the baby, could cause harm. Because these drugs are used for only very severe conditions, it is usually more important for the mother to take the drug than it is for her to nurse her baby. Generally, therefore, breastfeeding should not be undertaken when these drugs are used. Occasionally, some short-acting chemotherapy drugs are given in intermittent regimens that may allow a woman to resume nursing after stopping temporarily.

Cough, cold, allergy, and asthma medications. The various drugs used for these respiratory conditions are often taken together in combination products. These combination products should generally be avoided during breastfeeding. Usually only one or two symptoms are really troublesome, and a single-ingredient product can treat them effectively. For example, hay fever and other allergies can be treated with an antihistamine alone, and a cough can be treated with a cough syrup that has only one or two active ingredients. Oral sustained-release products should be avoided. Common sore throat lozenges (such as *Sucrets*, *Chloraseptic*, and *Hall's*) are safe to use. Drugs taken as nasal sprays or by inhaler reach the milk in lesser quantities than those taken orally and pose little risk of harm to the nursing infant.

Antihistamines. Antihistamines are used in many products for allergy, colds, coughs, and inducing sleep, although their use for colds is not justified. Antihistamines can reach the infant through breast milk in amounts large enough to cause drowsiness or fussiness. High doses of antihistamines, particularly when in combination with a decongestant or very soon after delivery, may decrease milk flow. Use no more than necessary to control symptoms; often a single dose at bedtime is sufficient. If you are planning to use an oral product, choose one with 2 milligrams or less of *chlorpheniramine* or *brompheniramine* per dose, or 25 milligrams or less of *diphenhydramine* per dose, and avoid sustained-release products. *Loratadine* and *fexofenadine* are well tolerated by infants and are preferred over the older sedating antihistamines. *Cetirizine* can cause drowsiness and may possibly affect lactation; it is not a good choice while nursing.

Most nonprescription medications for motion sickness, such as *dimenhydrinate* and *meclizine*, are also antihistamines. One or two doses of these medications should have no effect on the infant other than temporary drowsiness. They are preferred over the *scopolamine* patch, which is more likely to suppress lactation.

Asthma inhalers and nasal inhalers. These may contain a bronchodilator (such as *albuterol*, *salmeterol*, or *ipratropium*) or a corticosteroid (such as *beclomethasone*, *fluticasone*, *flunisolide*, or *triamcinolone*). All of these reach the mother's bloodstream in very low levels, so levels in milk also are low. Try to avoid swallowing excess medication after using an inhaler, because swallowed medication can enter the blood from the intestinal tract and reach the milk. Rinse your mouth and throat, and spit out the excess medication.

Cough medicines. The two most common drugs are *guaiafenesin* and *dextromethorphan*, both of which are safe to use during breastfeeding.

Decongestants. Nasal sprays (*Afrin, Nostrilla*) are preferable to oral drugs, especially if the baby is a newborn. A salt-water spray (such as *Ocean*) or rinse is quite safe to use during nursing. Oral decongestants can cause agitation or fussiness in the infant, and, most important, they can decrease the milk supply and might eventually cause the milk to dry up. The risk is greatest during the first six weeks after delivery. If you are planning to use an oral product, choose one with 30 milligrams or less of *pseudoephedrine* per dose; avoid sustained-release and products with other ingredients.

Theophylline. Aminophylline and other theophylline products have been well studied in breast milk. Occasionally they can cause jitteriness or fussiness in infants, usually newborns. In general, these drugs are acceptable during nursing.

Diuretics. Large doses of diuretics, especially the most potent ones and those that are long-acting, can decrease milk production; in fact, diuretics have been used for this purpose. Their passage into milk has not been well studied, but the amounts received by infants are likely to be small. These small amounts might in rare instances cause a rash or other allergic reaction in the infant.

Chlorthalidone. This very long-acting diuretic should not be used during breastfeeding, because it suppresses lactation. It might also accumulate in the infant.

Furosemide. This potent drug has been used to suppress lactation. It should be used cautiously, in small doses.

Hydrochlorothiazide. Given once daily in usual doses, this drug appears safe. Larger doses given several times daily have been used to suppress lactation.

Other thiazides. Long-acting thiazides should be avoided during breast-feeding.

Spironolactone. This drug appears in insignificant amounts in milk.

Ergot alkaloids

Bromocriptine has been used after birth to suppress lactation, but it is no longer approved for this use because it can be severely toxic to the mother.

Cabergoline. This potent, long-acting drug can stop lactation after a single dose. Don't use it if you intend to nurse your baby.

Ergonovine and methylergonovine. These drugs are often given to mothers right after delivery to diminish uterine bleeding. Methylergonovine is preferred, because ergonovine can suppress lactation. With the usual doses and the normal length of treatment, these drugs cause no problems in the breastfed newborn infant. Large amounts, however, might cause nausea, vomiting, and diarrhea in the baby. These effects may occasionally occur when the drugs are used beyond the immediate postpartum period.

See also ergotamine, in "Arthritis, Pain, and Migraine Medications," page 263.

Gastrointestinal drugs. Many of the drugs in this class act in the stomach and intestine and are not absorbed into the bloodstream; they cannot, therefore, appear in milk. Other gastrointestinal drugs are absorbed and can affect the infant through breast milk. If a choice exists, choose a drug that is not absorbed.

Antacids. These drugs are poorly absorbed and are safe to use during breastfeeding.

Antidiarrheals. Loperamide and *diphenoxylate* have not been well studied, but one or two small doses daily should pose little risk to the nursing infant. *Bismuth subsalicylate* is best avoided because of the large amount of absorbable salicylate it contains. Salicylate in large amounts can be toxic to the baby.

Domperidone. This drug is used to stimulate intestinal movement. Like metoclopramide, it has been used to increase milk production. It appears to be less likely to cause depression in the mother than metoclopramide. Domperidone, however, is not licensed for use in the United States.

Histamine H-2 antagonists. During breastfeeding, *famotidine* and *nizatidine* are the preferred drugs in this class, especially if the baby is young, because they reach the mother's milk in the lowest amounts. Larger amounts of *ranitidine* enter milk, but it is often used in newborn infants, so it is safe to take while breastfeeding. *Cimetidine* is the least desirable of this group. If your baby is older and is no longer nursing at night, you can take a single daily dose of any of these drugs at bedtime just after the baby's last feeding.

Laxatives. Many of the more potent laxatives are absorbed into the bloodstream; they have caused increased frequency of stools in breastfed infants. *Aloe, cascara,* and *senna* can affect the breastfed infant if taken in high doses but are safe to use occasionally in small amounts. Bulk-forming laxatives such as bran and other fibers (*Metamucil, Fibercon*) are not absorbed into the bloodstream and are therefore safe to use. Likewise, stool-softening agents such as *docusate* are not absorbable. *Bisacodyl* is a stronger laxative, but it is not absorbed into the bloodstream, either. Saline cathartics such as *Phospho-Soda* and *milk of magnesia* are poorly absorbed and do not affect the composition of milk. *Glycerin* suppositories are also safe to use.

Mesalamine derivatives. Diarrhea and bloody stools have occurred on rare occasions in infants of mothers using one of the mesalamine derivatives, *mesalamine, olsalazine,* or *sulfasalazine.* These drugs may be used during nursing, but the baby must be closely observed for side effects.

Metoclopramide. This medication is used to stimulate intestinal movement. It has also been used to increase the milk supply in women who are producing insufficient quantities of milk, such as mothers of premature or sick infants, and in adoptive mothers. Metoclopramide does not appear to harm the infant if it is used for two weeks or less. Since metoclopramide may cause or worsen depression, however, it should not be used by women with a history of depression, and it should not be used for long periods of time.

Proton-pump inhibitors. Omeprazole is the only drug of this type that has been studied during nursing, and information about it is limited. Levels in milk appear to be very low. No harm has occurred in breastfed infants whose mothers have taken this drug; in fact, omeprazole is given directly to infants. *Esomeprazole* is a form of omeprazole and so is probably just as safe. Since other drugs in this class (*lansoprazole, pantoprazole, rabeprazole*) have not been studied during breastfeeding, omeprazole is preferable for now. However, lansoprazole has been used safely in infants, so it is probably acceptable also.

Sucralfate. This drug acts locally in the mother's intestinal tract and poses no harm to the breastfed infant.

Heart and blood pressure drugs. These drugs are not often used in women of breastfeeding age, and information about them is therefore limited. Very little is known, in particular, about newer agents in the group.

ACE inhibitors. Benazepril, captopril, enalapril, and *quinapril* are safe to use while nursing. No other drugs in this class have been studied during breastfeeding.

Amiodarone. This drug has caused low thyroid levels and delayed growth in a breastfed infant. A few other infants whose mothers have taken the drug have been breastfed without harm. Using this medication while nursing requires close monitoring of your baby, including tests of thyroid function.

Angiotensin-2 blockers. There is no experience with any drugs in this class during nursing or in infants. It is best to avoid these drugs until more is known.

Beta blockers. The oldest drug in the group, *propranolol,* is also the best studied and safest. *Metoprolol* and *labetalol* are safe to use, too. These drugs reach the milk in insignificant amounts.

The long-acting drugs, such as *acebutolol, atenolol, nadolol, sotalol,* and *timolol,* reach the milk in higher quantities and also have a greater tendency to accumulate in the infant's bloodstream. These should be avoided during breastfeeding, especially with a newborn.

Calcium-channel blockers. Information on *diltiazem, nitrendipine,* and *verapamil* is limited, but amounts in milk do not appear to be large enough to affect nursing infants. *Nifedipine* has been well studied and is safe to use; it is sometimes used to treat painful nipple vasospasm caused by Raynaud's phenomenon.

Clonidine. Clonidine and the related drug *guanfacine* may affect milk production in complex and somewhat unpredictable ways. They might either increase or decrease milk production. Clonidine reaches the milk in high levels, and breastfed infants have blood concentrations of the drug approaching those of their mothers. Other blood pressure drugs are preferred, but if these drugs can't be avoided, they should be used with caution during breastfeeding.

Digoxin. This drug is excreted into milk in only small amounts. It can be used safely during lactation.

Hydralazine. Amounts of this drug excreted into milk are small. Hydralazine can be used safely during lactation.

Methyldopa. Amounts of this drug excreted into milk are small. Methyldopa has been used safely during nursing for many years.

Procainamide. Amounts that reach the milk are small. This drug appears safe to use while nursing.

Reserpine. Because this drug can cause nasal stuffiness in infants, it should be avoided during lactation.

Herbals.
There is a mistaken tendency to think that because herbal medications are "natural" they are never toxic. This is not true. Each herbal product must be evaluated individually according to its own merits and risks. Unfortunately, almost none of these products has been studied during lactation, and very few have been studied in infants. Because these medications are poorly regulated in the United States, the quality and amounts of ingredients and even the ingredients themselves can vary widely from batch to batch and from one manufacturer to another. Additionally, because plant products may contain dozens of chemicals that can cause allergies, they may be more likely than conventional medications to cause problems like asthma and skin rashes in an infant or lead to plant allergies later in his life. For all these reasons, using herbal products during nursing is somewhat risky. Information on some of the most commonly used herbals is listed here.

Blessed thistle. This herb is sometimes used to stimulate lactation, but no scientific studies confirm its effectiveness. In fact, there have been no studies at all of the herb's effects during lactation. Blessed thistle appears to be fairly safe, but allergic reactions have been reported.

Echinacea. There have been no studies of this herb during lactation. Although it is often used to prevent colds, scientific studies have shown it to be of no benefit.

Fenugreek. Most commonly used as a spice, fenugreek seeds are often used to stimulate lactation and increase milk supply. Although there have been no scientific studies on this use, it is considered a safe food substance; it is used as the flavoring in artificial maple syrup. Fenugreek can lower the blood sugar, so diabetic women should not use it without consulting a physician. Allergic reactions have also been reported.

Ginkgo biloba. There have been no studies on the use of ginkgo during lactation. Side effects are generally mild, but allergic skin reactions have occurred, and these could occur in the nursing infant of a mother who uses gingko.

Kava kava. There have been no studies on the use of kava kava during lactation. Chronic use can cause dry, discolored, flaky skin and muscle weakness. Kava kava has also caused liver damage in some users. Although we don't know whether enough is transmitted through breast milk to cause these effects in the nursing infant, kava kava is best avoided during breastfeeding.

Saint John's wort. Colic, drowsiness, and lethargy have occurred in breastfed infants whose mothers have taken Saint John's wort, a popular remedy for depression. In fair-skinned persons, Saint John's wort may cause allergic skin reactions with exposure to light. Besides, the wisdom of self-medication for a serious condition such as depression is doubtful. Saint John's wort should certainly be avoided during lactation.

Yerba mate. This herb, found in some diet products, is a source of caffeine, which in large amounts can cause fussiness in breastfed infants. Be careful not to use yerba mate along with coffee or caffeinated soft drinks.

Hormones. Several classes of drugs fall into the category of hormones, and each class must be considered separately. Because hormones are potent agents that might affect a baby's development, it is of paramount importance to consider both the dosage and the duration of therapy.

Antidiabetes drugs. Acarbose is not absorbed from the mother's intestinal tract, so its use is safe during breastfeeding. *Insulin* therapy for diabetes mellitus restores insulin that is normally produced in the body. A diabetic mother using insulin may breastfeed. For a few days to a few weeks after giving birth, though, she may need to reduce her insulin dose below the dose she took before pregnancy. Since insulin is inactivated in the baby's stomach, none that enters the milk will be absorbed into the infant's bloodstream. *Metformin* is found in small enough amounts in milk that it is unlikely to affect the breastfed infant. The small amount of information available on the *sulfonylureas, glyburide, tolbutamide,* and *chlorpropamide,* indicates that they can be used during breastfeeding. Other oral sulfonylureas and *thiazolidinediones (pioglitazone, rosiglitazone)* have not been studied during breastfeeding.

Antithyroid agents. Breastfeeding during treatment with *propylthiouracil* is safe. *Methimazole* in daily doses of 20 milligrams or less may also be safe, but larger doses may adversely affect the infant. With any antithyroid drug, monitoring of the infant's blood for adequate thyroid function may be necessary.

Bone-marrow stimulants. Epoetin alfa is an injection that stimulates the production of red blood cells. Although small amounts enter breast milk, this drug is not absorbed from the infant's intestinal tract and so has no effect on the nursing infant. *Filgrastim* and *sargramostim* are similar to epoetin alfa, but they stimulate the production of white rather than red blood cells. The baby cannot absorb them from breast milk. All of these drugs are safe to use during breastfeeding.

Clomiphene. This synthetic hormone-like drug affects the activity of estrogen in the body and stimulates ovulation. There is no information on the drug during nursing. Because it could have serious adverse consequences on the sexual maturation of your infant, and because it could remain in your body and milk for weeks, you should stop nursing if you take it.

Contraceptives. Hormonal contraceptives are second to barrier methods as a safe choice for birth control during breastfeeding. Hormonal contraceptives can be divided into two categories: combination and progestin-only. Since the combination products contain estrogen, they can decrease milk production and cause early weaning, although any long-term effects on a baby's growth and development have not been found. Included among the combination contraceptives is the vaginal ring (NuvaRing), the contraceptive patch (OrthoEvra) and one injection product (Lunelle). It is best not to use a combination contraceptive during breastfeeding unless you intend to stop nursing soon. If you plan to use hormonal contraception, a progestin-only oral product such as *norethindrone (Micronor, Nor-Q.D.)* or *norethynodrel (Ovrette)* or a progestin product given by injection (*Depo-Provera*) or implantation (*Norplant*) is preferable. Some intrauterine devices (IUDs) release small amounts of progesterone or progestin (for example, Progestasert and Mirena); these are considered as safe as other progestin-only contraceptives. There are two types of emergency or "morning-after" birth-control products. One is essentially a higher dose of a combination contraceptive (Preven); the other (*Plan B*) is a high dose of progestin-only contraceptive. The short duration of exposure to morning-after contraceptives should not adversely affect your infant and should have only a temporary effect on lactation. Progestin-only contraceptive injections or implants are sometimes given within a few days after birth, but we know little about the effects of this practice on breastfeeding and the breastfed infant. Because hormonal contraceptives might interfere with the establishment of lactation or affect the newborn infant, you should probably wait at least six weeks after the birth before starting on any hormonal contraceptive.

Corticosteroids. Drugs in this category include *cortisone, methylprednisolone, prednisone,* and *triamcinolone.* Low doses and short courses of therapy (up to two weeks) appear to pose no harm to the breastfed infant. Some breastfeeding mothers have taken 8 milligrams prednisolone or methylprednisolone for months without harming their infants. Of concern are long courses of treatment (several weeks to months) with moderate to large doses. Although only a small fraction of each dose appears in breast milk, no one knows what these amounts might do to the developing infant.

DHEA. This hormone-like drug is available without a prescription. There have been no studies of DHEA during lactation, but it is a chemical normally present in the body. Women of childbearing age, however, have near maximum amounts in their body. Because additional DHEA taken as a supplement might affect the infant or suppress lactation, you should avoid taking this drug during nursing.

Estrogens. Estrogens have been used after birth to suppress lactation, but because they are sometimes toxic they are no longer used this way. Estrogen products such as *Premarin* and *Estrace* can probably interfere with lactation after oral or vaginal administration.

Progesterone. This natural hormone is sometimes given in suppositories for premenstrual syndrome. It is also found in one type of intrauterine device, or IUD, for birth control (*Progestasert*). Amounts of progesterone that appear in breast milk are small, and they are not absorbed by the infant.

Thyroid. Thyroid products have one major, valid use—to replace thyroid that is lacking in the bloodstream. When a woman takes proper doses, her thyroid levels become approximately normal. Thyroid replacement, therefore, poses no risks to the breastfed infant. Large daily doses of thyroid hormone (more than about 100 micrograms of *levothyroxine*) may affect the infant, however.

Immunosuppressants and immunomodulators

Azathioprine. A few mothers have safely breastfed their infants while taking azathioprine following kidney transplantation.

Cyclosporine. Limited experience indicates that cyclosporine may be safe to take while nursing, but the infant should be carefully monitored, possibly with blood tests.

Glatiramer. No information exists on the use of this drug during breast-feeding. Because the baby is unlikely to absorb it from breast milk, however, harmful effects are unlikely.

Interferons. Several interferon drugs are available. Because they are large molecules, they are unlikely to pass into milk and affect the breastfed infant, as was found to be the case in studies of three breastfeeding women who were taking *interferon alfa.* Also, these drugs are active only when given by injection, so any interferon that reaches the milk has little or no effect on the infant. There is no information on the effects of *interferon beta* during breastfeeding, but this drug is likely to be similar to interferon alfa in its passage into milk and safety during breastfeeding.

Tacrolimus. There has been minimal experience with tacrolimus during nursing. Amounts in milk appear small, but the infant should be carefully monitored, possibly with blood tests.

Lipid-lowering drugs. None of the cholesterol-lowering drugs have been studied during nursing. Because cholesterol is essential for the proper development of the infant's brain and nervous system, cholesterol-lowering drugs that can enter the milk should not be taken during nursing. The most potent and common of these drugs, called "statins," include *atorvastatin, fluvastatin, lovastatin, pravastatin, rosuvastatin,* and *simvastatin.* Other cholesterol-lowering drugs that can enter the milk are the "fibrates," including *fenofibrate* and *gemfibrozil.* All of these drugs should be avoided during nursing. *Cholestyramine, colestipol,* and *colesevelam* are resins that work only in the mother's intestinal tract; they can be safely used during nursing. It is unclear whether *ezetimibe* or high-dose *niacin* can affect the nursing infant.

Muscle relaxants. Most of these drugs have not been studied during nursing. Muscle relaxants taken by mouth, such as *carisoprodol, chlorzoxazone, diazepam,* and *methocarbamol,* are sedatives and can be expected to cause drowsiness in breastfed infants. *Cyclobenzaprine* probably doesn't reach high levels in milk, but it has not been studied during nursing. In general, it is best to avoid these drugs while breastfeeding, if possible. Taking ibuprofen or acetaminophen along with mild to moderate exercise will usually ease muscle spasms and pain as well as muscle relaxants could.

Nonmedical drugs. Since drugs used for nontherapeutic purposes are not essential to the well-being of the mother, and since their effects on a breast-fed infant are often unknown, their use is generally discouraged. Additionally, even small amounts can cause positive drug tests in your infant's urine, which with some drugs could lead to legal problems.

Alcohol. Alcohol readily passes into the milk. Large amounts of alcoholic beverages consumed over a short time can make a baby drunk and can inhibit the let-down reflex. Heavy daily drinking can lead to hormonal imbalances in a breastfed infant, and even small to moderate amounts of alcohol taken daily or nearly every day while nursing appear to cause delayed muscular development and coordination in infants, although the severity of this problem depends on the amount of alcohol used. Right after you drink an alcoholic beverage, your infant may suck more but consume up to 25 percent less milk; he will make up for the lack later in the day if you take no more alcohol. An occasional alcoholic beverage probably does not pose a serious danger to the infant, but it is prudent to wait at least two hours per drink before nursing and to refrain from daily or near-daily alcohol use.

Amphetamines. Amphetamine and *methamphetamine* ("crystal," "crystal meth") have not been formally studied during nursing. However, they are potent stimulants. Breastfeeding mothers who take these drugs often have fussy infants who cry a lot, cannot be comforted easily, and do not sleep well. Amphetamines probably also inhibit the mother's milk production. These drugs should not be used during nursing; if they are, the mother should stop nursing for 24 to 48 hours after taking them.

Caffeine. Low to moderate intake of beverages containing caffeine is unlikely to cause problems in the infant, since the amount of caffeine that reaches the milk is usually small. But very high caffeine intake (more than 10 cups of coffee per day, for example) can make the baby jittery and agitated.

Cocaine. Cocaine is extremely toxic to infants because they metabolize it very slowly. Great agitation and continuous crying are often noted in breastfed infants of cocaine users; some of these babies have had convulsions. Cocaine must be avoided during nursing. A mother should stop breastfeeding for at least 24 to 48 hours after taking cocaine.

Hallucinogens. Information is lacking on the effects of these drugs during breastfeeding; however, levels in milk should be low by the time the mother has stopped feeling the effects of the drug.

Marijuana. There are few reports of the effects of marijuana in breastfed babies. After a single use, marijuana levels in milk are apparently low, but the active component of the drug is very fat-soluble and can build up in the body with daily or near-daily use. Because milk has a high fat content, marijuana levels are probably high in the milk of chronic users. Note, too, that an infant in the same room with a smoker will breathe in significant quantities of marijuana. Breastfed infants whose mothers use marijuana heavily have sometimes shown delayed muscular development and coordination. Marijuana and its metabolites are detectable in the urine of breastfed infants whose mothers use marijuana.

Narcotics. Large doses can cause narcotic effects and addiction in breastfed infants. Narcotic addicts should not breastfeed; however, mothers on methadone maintenance can often breastfeed their infants safely. *See also* "Arthritis, Pain, and Migraine Medications," page 263.

Phencyclidine (PCP). Large amounts of this drug have been measured in the breast milk of users. PCP must be entirely avoided during breastfeeding.

Smoking and nicotine. Nicotine from smoking tobacco appears in breast milk. Other toxic substances in smoke probably reach the milk as well. Smoking interferes with lactation, causing smokers to stop nursing and start supplementing sooner than nonsmokers. If you smoke, your infant is likely to have more colic symptoms and respiratory infections than if you did not smoke. Additionally, although breastfeeding reduces the risk of sudden infant death syndrome (SIDS), smoking negates this advantage. If you can't stop smoking while you are nursing, you should (1) decrease your smoking as much as possible, (2) avoid smoking just before nursing, (3) avoid smoking in the same room with your baby, and (4) cover your regular clothing while you smoke and remove the covering before breastfeeding. Amounts of nicotine in the breast milk of women using nicotine patches appear to be about the same as that found in the milk of smokers. Still, using a nicotine patch or nicotine chewing gum during breastfeeding is safer than smoking.

Psychotherapeutic agents. For many of these drugs, little is known about their excretion into milk or their effects on infants. Undertake nursing with caution if you are using one of these drugs.

Major tranquilizers. These drugs include the *phenothiazines*, such as *chlorpromazine, thioridazine, trifluoperazine, perphenazine,* and *fluphenazine*; the closely related *thioxanthenes*, such as *thiothixene*; the *butyrophenones*, such as *haloperidol*; and the newer "atypical" drugs such as *clozapine, olanzapine, quetiapine, risperidone,* and *ziprasidone*. Small amounts of these drugs appear in breast milk, and occasionally they have caused drowsiness in breastfed infants. Long-term effects on the infant are not well known. One study found no altered development in infants exposed to one of these drugs through breast milk; however, use of two of the drugs together had an adverse effect on an infant's development. Nursing is not recommended during *clozapine* therapy because harmful side effects may occur in the infant.

Antidepressants. Untreated postpartum depression can have serious and long-lasting effects on an infant's growth and development, so treatment is essential. Medications are often used in such treatment. Small amounts of tricyclic antidepressants such as *amitriptyline, imipramine, nortriptyline,* and *desipramine* do not seem to affect the growth and development of the breastfed infant. Some of the more sedating tricyclic antidepressants, such as *doxepin*, could make a baby drowsy and should be avoided. Nortriptyline appears to be the safest and best studied of all the tricyclic antidepressants; it is found only in small amounts in milk, and little or none reaches the infant's bloodstream. If possible, take tricyclic antidepressants in the evening after the final nursing session of the day to minimize the amount that your baby receives.

Fluoxetine appears in milk in higher amounts than most other antidepressants; it is very long-acting; and side effects (colic, fussiness, and drowsiness) have been reported in breastfed babies during the use of this drug. It should be avoided if the baby is less than one month old, but an older infant can probably tolerate it better. If fluoxetine is needed, the benefits of breastfeeding probably outweigh the risks to the infant, but watch her carefully for side effects.

Citalopram is found in relatively large amounts in milk, and it may cause drowsiness in the infant, so it is best avoided, especially with a newborn. *Escitalopram* is a form of citalopram that is taken in a lower dose; it is preferred over citalopram.

Other drugs in the same class as fluoxetine and citalopram are *fluvoxamine, paroxetine,* and *sertraline.* These are found in lower amounts in milk and are shorter-acting than fluoxetine. Sertraline and paroxetine are the best studied and do not seem to affect nursing infants in the short or long run. They are good choices when an antidepressant is needed during nursing.

Bupropion has been studied in a small number of mother-infant pairs, and it appears not to have harmed the nursing infants. Limited data indicate that *trazodone* is also probably safe during nursing, but watch for excessive drowsiness if you are nursing a newborn.

Nefazodone has not been well studied, but it has caused drowsiness and poor feeding in one newborn infant, so this drug is best avoided if you are nursing a newborn.

Venlafaxine is found in relatively high amounts in milk. Experience with it during breastfeeding is very limited, but no side effects have been seen in nursing infants. If possible, avoid this drug if you are nursing a newborn.

The monoamine oxidase inhibitors, *phenelzine* and *tranylcypromine,* are very potent drugs and should not be used while breastfeeding.

Other antidepressants, such as *amoxapine* and *maprotiline,* have been less well studied, so no judgment can be made about their safety.

Lithium. This drug sometimes reaches breast milk in high levels. It can accumulate in the bloodstream and cause side effects in a premature or newborn infant or one who becomes dehydrated due to diarrhea or a viral illness. A healthy infant may be breastfed during lithium therapy, but careful monitoring—including, in some cases, measuring his lithium blood level—is essential. If your infant becomes ill for any reason while you're taking lithium, stop breastfeeding and contact your physician.

Radiologic diagnostic agents. A number of compounds are used in the X-ray diagnosis of various conditions. These compounds fall into three categories: MRI contrast agents, radio-opaque contrast agents, and radioactive agents. The radiologist administering these tests will probably have guidelines on breastfeeding with the specific agents. X-rays of your teeth or bones pose no hazard to your breastfed infant.

MRI contrast agents. Gadodiamide, gadopentetate, gadoteridol, and *gadoversetamide* contain *gadolinium* rather than iodine and are relatively safe and rapidly eliminated. There appears to be no need to stop nursing for any length of time after receiving one of these agents.

Radio-opaque agents. These are generally compounds that contain iodine, but they vary in the amount of iodine that can pass into milk. Many are short-acting, have no free iodine, or both, and therefore pose little risk to the infant. Others require that the mother stop nursing for several hours after use.

Radioactive agents. Breastfeeding must be stopped for a time after most of these agents are administered. The period varies depending on the agent and the dose given; a few of these agents persist in breast milk for so long that complete weaning of the baby is necessary. For nursing mothers with overactive thyroid glands, the most commonly prescribed of these agents are *iodine-123* (for diagnosis) and *iodine-131* (for treatment). Although iodine-123 is eliminated in two to three days, it leaves the long-lasting by-product *iodine-124.* Experts disagree about the safety of these drugs, but it seems prudent to stop nursing the infant permanently after using them (you can breastfeed future babies, though). *Technetium (pertechnetate)* is a suitable alternative for diagnostic use. After exposure to some of these agents your body could give off significant amounts of radiation, particularly at close range. This means that not only will you have to stop breastfeeding temporarily, but you may not be able to hold your baby for some time, since doing so would expose her to significant radiation.

Sedatives and sleep medications. Several types of drugs are included in this category. Although all of them can make an infant drowsy, some are more likely to do so than others. The drugs also differ in how long they persist in the body, which affects their tendency to accumulate in the infant.

Barbiturates. Drugs in this class include *amobarbital, butalbital, pentobarbital, phenobarbital, secobarbital,* and others. All of them occasionally cause drowsiness in breastfed infants; phenobarbital is the most likely to do so. None of these drugs are particularly hazardous to the baby, however, unless she becomes so drowsy that she nurses less.

Benzodiazepines. Of all sedative drugs, these are the most frequently used. They include *alprazolam, chlordiazepoxide, diazepam, flurazepam, lorazepam, oxazepam, triazolam,* and others. Although these drugs are safe in adults, newborn infants do not readily metabolize them; the long-acting drugs in the group accumulate in the infant's body. This may make the baby drowsy, and, in some cases, may interfere with the binding of bilirubin in the bloodstream. These problems are accentuated in premature and newborn babies. Preferable benzodiazepines are short-acting and reach breast milk in lesser amounts, and are therefore unlikely to cause drowsiness. Safer benzodiazepines include *oxazepam*, *lorazepam*, and *triazolam*.

Two sleeping medications similar to the benzodiazepines are *zaleplon* and *zolpidem*. These are very short-acting and appear in milk in very small amounts, so they can be used while nursing.

Buspirone. No information exists on this drug during lactation. It is best avoided during nursing.

Chloral hydrate. Though old, this drug is still used sometimes. It has caused drowsiness in infants, but it is probably safe for occasional use. *Dichloralphenazone*, which is in *Midrin*, releases chloral hydrate in the mother's body and can cause drowsiness in the breastfed infant.

Over-the-counter sleep medications. Most of these contain *diphenhydramine*. The general precautions for the sedating antihistamines apply (see "Cough, Cold, Allergy, and Asthma Medications," page 265).

Iodine and iodide. Use of *povidone iodine*, especially as a douche, but even on the skin, can result in high iodine blood levels in the mother. Iodine in the body of a breastfeeding woman becomes concentrated in milk and subsequently in the infant's thyroid gland, where it might possibly cause abnormal thyroid function; iodide rashes have also occurred in breastfed infants. Iodides should not be used during lactation. See also "Radioopaque Agents," page 277.

Vaccines and skin tests. Smallpox is the only vaccine given to mothers that is known to pose a hazard to breastfed infants. Killed vaccines, including *diphtheria, hepatitis A* and *B, injectable influenza, injectable polio,* and *tetanus vaccines*, are inactive in breast milk. Live vaccines are occasionally transmitted through breast milk; with the exception of smallpox, they do not endanger the baby. Live vaccines include *inhaled influenza, measles, mumps, oral polio, rubella, smallpox, oral typhoid,* and *varicella*. The U.S. Centers for Disease Control states that, with the exception of smallpox, no vaccination should be withheld from a woman or delayed because she is breastfeeding. Skin tests such as the one for tuberculosis are also considered safe.

Weight-loss products. Excessive weight loss during lactation should be avoided, because many fat-soluble environmental contaminants (such as some insecticides) are stored in body fat. When body fat is lost rapidly, contaminants are released into the bloodstream and appear in the fat of breast milk in larger-than-usual amounts. In addition, some weight loss agents can affect infants directly or lessen the milk supply. *Chromium picolinate*, however, is probably safe in doses of 200 micrograms or less daily.

Many weight-loss products contain vitamins that may also be in multivitamin products prescribed by your physician. If you take both products your vitamin intake may be excessive.

INDEX TO COMMON DRUGS

Each brand name is listed in capital letters; the corresponding generic name is given after it. All generic names that do not appear as headings in the text are followed here by cross-references to the relevant sections. The names of combination products are followed by lists of the ingredients they contain; see the separate entry for each ingredient. Not all brands are listed, so if you can't find the name of a particular product in this list, look under the generic name of its ingredient or ingredients.

References

American Academy of Pediatrics. "Report on the Assessment of Scientific Evidence Relating to Infant-Feeding Practices and Infant Health." *Pediatrics* 74 (1984).

———. "Policy Statement: Breastfeeding and the Use of Human Milk." *Pediatrics* 100 (1997): 1035–1039.

Auerbach, Kathleen G. "Employed Breastfeeding Mothers: Problems They Encounter." *Birth* 11 (1984): 17–20.

Auerbach, Kathleen G., and Laurence Gartner. "Breastfeeding and Human Milk: Their Association with Jaundice in the Neonate." *Clinics in Perinatology* 14 (1987), 89–107.

Auerbach, Kathleen G., and E. Guss. "Maternal Employment and Breastfeeding: A Study of 567 Women's Experiences." *American Journal of Disease in Childhood* 138 (1984): 958–960.

Ballard, Jeanne L., et al. "Ankyloglossia: Assessment, Incidence, and Effect of Frenuloplasty on the Breastfeeding Dyad." *Pediatrics* 110 (2002): 62–68.

Bauer, G., et al. "Breastfeeding and Cognitive Development of Three Year Old Children." *Psychology Report* 68 (1991): 1218.

Bishop, N., M. McGraw, and N. Ward. "Aluminum in Infant Formulas." *Lancet* 1 (1989): 490.

Brazelton, T. Berry. *Infants and Mothers: Differences in Development.* Rev. ed. New York: Delta/Seymour Lawrence, 1983.

Brewster, Dorothy Patricia. *You Can Breastfeed Your Baby ... Even in Special Situations.* Emmaus, Penn.: Rodale Press, 1979.

Brown, Marie Scott, and Joan T. Hurlock. "Preparation of the Breast for Breastfeeding." *Nursing Research* 24 (1975): 448–451.

Byers, T., et al. "Lactation and Breast Cancer: Evidence for a Negative Association in Pre-Menopausal Women." *American Journal of Epidemiology* 121 (1985): 664–674.

Davis, M. K., D. A. Savitz, and B. I. Graubard. "Infant Feeding and Childhood Cancer." *Lancet* 2 (1988): 365–368.

DeCarvalho, M., M. Hall, and D. Harvey. "Effects of Water Supplementation on Physiological Jaundice in Breast-fed Babies." *Archives of Disease in Childhood* 56 (1981): 568–569.

Ehrenkranz, R., and B. Ackerman. "Metoclopromide Effect on Faltering Milk Production by Mothers of Premature Infants." *Pediatrics* 78 (1986): 614–620.

Elias, Marjorie F., et al. "Sleep/Wake Patterns of Breastfed Infants in the First 2 Years of Life." *Pediatrics* 77 (1986): 322–329.

Ferber, Richard. *Solve Your Child's Sleep Problems: The Complete Practical Guide for Parents.* New York: Simon and Schuster, 1985.

Frantz, Kittie B., Paul M. Fleiss, and Ruth A. Lawrence. "Management of the Slow-Gaining Breastfed Baby." *Keeping Abreast Journal* 3 (1978): 287–308.

Friedland, G., and R. Klein. "Transmission of the Human Immunodeficiency Virus." *New England Journal of Medicine* 317 (1987): 1125–1135.

Gwinn, M. L., et al. "Pregnancy, Breastfeeding, and Oral Contraceptives and the Risk of Epithelial Ovarian Cancer." *Journal of Clinical Epidemiology* 43 (1990): 559–568.

Hahn-Zoric, M., et al. "Antibody Responses to Parenteral and Oral Vaccines Are Impaired by Conventional and Low Protein Formulas as Compared to Breastfeeding." *Acta Paediatrica Scandanavica* 79 (1990): 1137–1142.

Huggins, Kathleen, et al. "Markers of Lactation Insufficiency: A Study of 34 Mothers." *Current Issues in Clinical Lactation* 1(2000): 25–35.

Huggins, Kathleen, and Sharon Billon. "Twenty Cases of Persistent Sore Nipples: Collaboration Between Lactation Consultant and Dermatologist." *Journal of Human Lactation* 9 (1993): 155–160.

Jensen, Rima. "Fenugreek—Overlooked But Not Forgotten." *UCLA Lactation Alumni Association Newsletter* 1 (1992): 2–3.

Karp, Harvey. "The 'Fourth Trimester': A Framework and Strategy for Understanding and Resolving Colic." *Contemporary Pediatrics* 21 (2004): 94–114.

Kavanaugh, Karen, et al. "Getting Enough: Mothers' Concerns about Breastfeeding a Preterm Infant after Discharge." *JOGNN* 24 (1995): 23–32.

Keating, J. P., G. J. Schears, and P. R. Dodge, "Oral Water Intoxication in Infants: An American Epidemic." *American Journal of Disease in Childhood* 145 (1991): 985–990.

Kennedy, Kathy, et al. "Consensus Statement on the Use of Breastfeeding as a Family Planning Method." *Contraception* 39 (1989): 477–496.

Koetting, C. A., and G. M. Wardlaw. "Wrist, Spine, and Hip Bone Density in Women with Variable Histories of Lactation." *American Journal of Clinical Nutrition* 48 (1988): 1479–1481.

Kowalchik, Claire, and William H. Hylton, eds. *Rodale's Illustrated Encyclopedia of Herbs*. Emmaus, Penn.: Rodale Press, 1987.

Labbok, M. H., and G. E. Hendershot. "Does Breastfeeding Protect Against Malocclusion? Analysis of the 1981 Child Health Supplement to the National Health Interview Survey." *American Journal of Preventative Medicine* 3 (1987): 227–232.

La Leche League International. *The Womanly Art of Breastfeeding*. Franklin Park, Ill.: La Leche League International, 1997.

Lawrence, Ruth A. *Breastfeeding: A Guide for the Medical Profession*. St. Louis: C.V. Mosby, 1994.

———. *A Review of the Medical Benefits and Contraindications to Breastfeeding in the United States*. Arlington, Virginia: National Center for Education in Maternal and Child Health, 1997.

Layde, P. M., et al. "The Independent Associations of Parity, Age of First Full-Term Pregnancy, and Duration of Breastfeeding with the Risk of Breast Cancer." *Journal of Clinical Epidemiology* 42 (1989): 963–973.

Livingstone, Varity, and L. Judy Stringer. "The Treatment of Staphyloccus Aureus Sore Nipples: A Randomized Comparative Study." *Journal of Human Lactation* 15, no. 3 (1999): 241–246.

Lucas, A., et al. "Breastmilk and Subsequent Intelligence Quotient in Children Born Preterm." *Lancet* 339 (1992): 261–264.

Mayer, E. J., et al. "Reduced Risk of IDDM among Breastfed Children." *Diabetes* 37 (1988): 1625–1632.

McJunkin, J. E., W. G. Bithoney, and M. C. McCormick. "Errors in Formula Concentration in an Outpatient Population." *Journal of Pediatrics* 111 (1987): 848–850.

McTiernan, A., and D. B. Thomas. "Evidence for a Protective Effect of Lactation on Risk of Breast Cancer in Young Women." *American Journal of Epidemiology* 124 (1986): 353–358.

Meier, Paula. "A Program to Support Breastfeeding in the High-Risk Nursery." *Perinatology/Neonatology* 4 (1980): 43–48.

———. *Professional Guide to Breastfeeding Premature Infants.* Columbus, Ohio: Abbott Laboratories, 1997.

Meier, Paula, and G. Anderson. "Responses of Small Preterm Infants to Bottle- and Breast-feeding." *Maternal-Child Nursing* 12 (1987): 97–105.

Merrett, T. G., et al. "Infant Feeding and Allergy: Twelve Month Prospective Study of 500 Babies Born in Allergic Families." *Annals of Allergy* 61 (1988): 13–20.

Michigan Department of Public Health. *Minutes of the Panel on Recommendations Relating to PBB and Nursing Mothers*, 1976.

Mitchell, E. A., et al. "Cot Death Supplement: Results from the First Year of the New Zealand Cot Death Study." *New Zealand Medical Journal* 104 (1991): 71–76.

Morrow-Tlucak, M., R. H. Haude, and C. B. Ernhart. "Breastfeeding and Cognitive Development in the First Two Years of Life." *Social Science Medicine* 26 (1988): 635–639.

Morse, Janice M., and Margaret J. Harrison. "Social Coercion for Weaning." *Journal of Nurse Midwifery* 32 (1987): 205–210.

Moscone, S. R., and M. J. Moore. "Breastfeeding During Pregnancy." *Journal of Human Lactation* 9 (1993): 83–88.

Neifert, M. R., and J. M. Seacat. "Contemporary Breastfeeding Management Clinics." *Perinatology* 12 (1995): 319–342.

Rickert, V. I., and C. Merle Johnson. "Reducing Nocturnal Awakening and Crying Episodes in Infants and Young Children: A Comparison Between Scheduled Awakenings and Systematic Ignoring." *Pediatrics* 81 (1988): 203–212.

Riordan, Janice. *A Practical Guide to Breastfeeding.* St. Louis: C.V. Mosby, 1983.

Riordan, Jan, and Kathleen Auerbach. *Breastfeeding and Human Lactation.* Boston: Jones and Bartlett, 1998.

Riordan, Jan, and Francine Nichols. "A Descriptive Study of Lactation Mastitis in Long-term Breastfeeding Women." *Journal of Human Lactation* 6, no. 2 (1990): 53–58.

Satter, Ellyn. *Child of Mine: Feeding with Love and Good Sense*. Palo Alto, Calif.: Bull Publishing, 1991.

Walker, Marsha. "A Fresh Look at the Risks of Artificial Infant Feeding." *Journal of Human Lactation* 9 (1993): 97–107.

Weintraub, R., G. Hams, M. Meerkin, and A. Rosenberg. "High Aluminum Content of Infant Milk Formulas." *Archives of Disease in Childhood* 61 (1986): 914–916.

Wickizer, Thomas M., Lawrence B. Brilliant, Richard Copeland, and Robert Tilden. "Polychlorinated Biphenyl Contamination of Nursing Mothers' Milk in Michigan." *American Journal of Public Health* 71 (1981): 132–137.

Woolridge, M. W., and Chloe Fisher. "Colic, 'Overfeeding,' and Symptoms of Lactose Malabsorption in the Breast-fed Baby: A Possible Artifact of Feed Management?" *Lancet* 2 (1988): 382–384.

Victora, C. G., et al. "Use of Pacifiers and Breastfeeding Duration." *Lancet* 341 (1993): 404–406.

Suggested
Supplemental Reading

Most of the books listed here are available in bookstores. If you can't find or order them locally, contact Cascade HealthCare Products or ICEA Bookcenter, both of which publish catalogs. Cascade and ICEA Bookcenter accept telephone orders.

Cascade HealthCare Products
(Birth and Life Bookstore)
1826 Northwest 18th Avenue
Portland, Oregon 97209
503-595-1720
800-443-9942 (orders only)

ICEA Bookcenter
P.O. Box 20048
Minneapolis, Minnesota 55420
952-854-8660
800-624-4934 (orders only)

La Leche League pamphlets are available by contacting—

La Leche League International
1400 North Meacham Road
Schaumburg, Illinois 60173
847-519-9585

Childbirth Graphics pamphlets are available by contacting—

Childbirth Graphics
P.O. Box 21207
Waco, Texas 76702
800-299-3366

Bumgarner, Norma Jane. *Mothering Your Nursing Toddler*. Shaumburg, Ill.: La Leche League International, 1982.

Danner, Sarah Coulter, and Edward R. Cerrutti. *Nursing Your Baby with a Cleft Palate or Cleft Lip*. Rochester, N.Y.: Childbirth Graphics, 1994. This pamphlet can be ordered for $2.00 from Childbirth Graphics.

Fraiberg, Selma H. *The Magic Years*. New York: Charles Scribner's Sons, 1959. A classic text on child development from infancy to six years.

Good, Judy. *The Diabetic Mother and Breastfeeding.* Shaumburg, Ill.: La Leche League International, 1987.

Gotsch, Gwen. *Breastfeeding a Baby with Down Syndrome.* Shaumburg, Ill.: La Leche League International, 1998.

Gromada, Karen. *Mothering Multiples.* Shaumburg, Ill.: La Leche League International, 1998.

Huggins, Kathleen, and Linda Ziedrich. *The Nursing Mother's Guide to Weaning.* Boston: Harvard Common Press, 1994.

Jones, Sandy. *Crying Baby, Sleepless Nights.* Boston: Harvard Common Press, 1992.

Karp, Harvey. *The Happiest Baby on the Block.* New York: Bantam Books, 2002.

Kleiman, Karen R., and Valerie D. Raskin. *This Isn't What I Expected: Overcoming Postpartum Depression.* New York: Bantam Books, 1994.

Pantley, Elizabeth. *The No-Cry Sleep Solution.* New York: Contemporary Books, 2002.

Robertson, Laurel, Carol Flinders, and Brian Ruppenthal. *The New Laurel's Kitchen.* Berkeley: Ten Speed Press, 1986.

Satter, Ellyn. *Child of Mine: Feeding with Love and Good Sense.* Expanded ed. Palo Alto, Calif.: Bull Publishing, 1991.

Thevenin, Tine. *The Family Bed: An Age Old Concept in Child Rearing.* Minneapolis: Tine Thevenin, 1976.

INDEX